TRUST
Yourself
to Transform
Your Body

Stacy—
Trust Yourself,
and you can
accomplish
anything
Laura K. Bryant

TRUST
Yourself
to Transform
Your Body

A Woman's Guide to Health and Weight Loss Without Diets

Laura K. Bryant, MA, CFT

Crimson Leaf Publishing
GURNEE, ILLINOIS

Crimson Leaf Publishing
P.O. Box 7836, Gurnee, IL 60031
E-mail: crimsonleafpub@sbcglobal.net
Web: www.crimsonleafpub.com

Although the author and publisher have made every effort to ensure the
accuracy and completeness of information contained in this book, we assume
no responsibility for errors, inaccuracies, omissions, or any inconsistency
herein. Any slights of people, places, or organizations are unintentional.

First printing 2005

ISBN 0-9753561-0-0   LCCN 2004092938

ATTENTION CORPORATIONS, UNIVERSITIES, COLLEGES, AND
PROFESSIONAL ORGANIZATIONS: Quantity discounts are available on
bulk purchases of this book for educational, gift purposes, or as premiums for
increasing magazine subscriptions or renewals. Special books or book excerpts
can also be created to fit specific needs. For information, please contact
Crimson Leaf Publishing, P.O. Box 7836, Gurnee, IL 60031;
crimsonleafpub@sbcglobal.net.

ABOUT THE AUTHOR

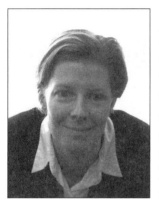 **Laura K. Bryant** holds a master's degree in clinical psychology. After years of being overweight and not feeling good about herself, she created her own fitness plan and succeeded in reaching and maintaining a healthy weight and lifestyle. She is a certified personal trainer and owns her own company designed to help women live phenomenally better lives. She has dedicated her career to helping inspire fitness and healthy living in others.

To Gregory Scott,
You never stop believing in me.
Thank you.

This publication contains the thoughts and opinions of its author. It is sold with the understanding that the publisher and author are not engaged in administering medical, psychological, or other professional services. If medical, psychological, or other assistance is required, please consult a competent professional. Individuals who are currently under a doctor's care should not change what they are eating or begin exercising until they have consulted with a physician. This book is not a substitute for medical or psychological advice or treatment. The purpose of this guide is to educate and inspire. The publisher and the author disclaim all responsibility for any loss, liability, or risk, personal or otherwise, that is caused as a consequence, directly or indirectly, of using or applying any information in this book.

ACKNOWLEDGMENTS

Thank you to my friends and family for all the support you provided and continue to provide. A special thanks to Niki Berlin, Lana Weiss Brown, Lori Chevrette, Sue Ehrhardt, George Foster, Jane Frederick, Jan Glover, Joan Goldner, Meagan Gottcent, Mara Gundrum, Tangela Johnson, Chris Lynch, Earl O'Kuly, James Orvis, Kati Powers, Dan Poynter, Jodie Rodgers, Richard E. Schell J.D., Tiana Sunshine Silva, Laura Slominski, Jill Stranczek, LuAnn Sullivan, Barbara Unser, and everyone at About Books, Inc. for their contributions to this work.

Finally, thank you to all the women who choose to make their health and well-being a priority. You inspire me every day.

CONTENTS

xi

It Is Possible

Whether you believe it now or whether you don't, you can lose weight and keep it off for a lifetime. You can feel good about yourself, your body, and the choices you make. You can be fit, strong, and self-assured. By picking up this book, you have taken the first step toward achieving these goals.

Not an Exact Science

What if I could tell you exactly what you needed to do to lose weight and maintain the loss? Would you do it? What if it meant working out at 4:30 every morning, when right now you can barely get out of bed by 7:00? What if it meant eliminating every food you associate with comfort, fun, and family? Or what if it involved biking for two hours every day? Would you do it then?

Diet and weight-loss "experts" act as if there is a secret formula for losing weight. That if you do exactly what they tell you to do, when, where, and how they tell you to do it, the pounds will just drop off. The piece these "experts" are missing is that each woman is different. Your needs, goals, and situation are different from any other woman's. Therefore, you require a customized plan.

While there are strategies that help the fitness effort, nothing is exact. Only you can determine what works best for you.

How This Book Is Organized

Each chapter of *Trust Yourself* takes you through a stage of the process necessary for success. The first chapter, "What If I Could Do It?" takes you through the feelings of doubt anyone has before starting something new, tells you what you need to know about diets and the diet industry, and asks that you make a commitment to yourself and to your body. The second chapter, "I Can Do It!" shows you how to change the way you think and act to get you where you want to be. Chapter three, "I Will Do It!" shows you step-by-step how to create the plan that will get you the results you want. The fourth chapter, "I Am Doing It!" discusses common obstacles, how to move past them, and how to create a lifelong health habit. The fifth chapter, "I Did It!" acknowledges all you have achieved, while asking you to achieve so much more.

Getting the Most from This Book

Here are some suggestions on how to best use *Trust Yourself*:

1. Take the suggestions in the book and make them your own. Adapt the ideas to your situation and needs. This process is all about determining what works best for you.

2. Keep an open mind. *Trust Yourself* challenges many of the messages you've heard and urges you to take full responsibility for your health. It asks you to try new things and to have faith in the process and in yourself.

3. Maintain your focus. Once you've made the commitment to yourself and to your health, focus on doing what it

takes to reach your goals. Use *Trust Yourself* to guide you through each stage of the process.

4. Educate yourself. Read *Trust Yourself* more than once. Read other books and newsletters on health and nutrition, hire fitness professionals, or attend classes. Only when you educate yourself can you truly make the best decisions. Look for other excellent resources at the back of this book and at www.trustyourselftotransform.com.

5. Do the written exercises. The exercises are there for a reason—to help you create your best plan possible and achieve the results you want. I urge you to do them all.

6. As you read, make notes, underline, highlight text, or fold down the pages. Make *Trust Yourself* yours.

You Can Do It

I know how hard it is to try something new, something different. If you've tried losing weight and have always gained it back, you wonder if it's even possible to keep it off. You believe less and less that you will ever reach your goal weight. You begin to believe you are destined to be fat.

This is not the case. You can reach and maintain a healthy weight. You can become stronger, fit, and more confident. You can change the way you feel about your body and yourself. Your body will respond when you treat it with the respect it deserves and make the decisions that are right for you. *Trust Yourself to Transform Your Body.*

CHAPTER 1

What If I Could Do It?

MAKING THE DECISION

Are You Willing to Do What It Takes?

Women who want to lose weight often spend a lot of time, effort, and money on diet books, foods, and pills. If you've done that in the past, it's time to stop. You wouldn't be reading this book if you'd gotten the results you wanted.

Consistently looking to diets and weight-loss gadgets for permanent weight loss means you're hoping for a quick fix, an easy way out. Reaching and maintaining a healthy weight takes living a healthy lifestyle. It takes dedication, and a belief in yourself and what you can accomplish. You must acknowledge, take responsibility for, and change the attitudes, thoughts,

> ...*until a person can say deeply and honestly "I am what I am today because of the choices I made yesterday" that person cannot say, "I choose otherwise."*
>
> —Stephen R. Covey

and behaviors that are responsible for where you are today. No diet, pill, or gadget can do this; only you can.

Women who try diet after diet question their ability to lose weight on their own. They think they need a pill or some diet to lose the weight. It is possible to reach a healthy weight and feel good about yourself and your body if you're willing to look inside and make the necessary changes. You can achieve your weight-loss goals on your own, without diets, pills, and gadgets.

WRITTEN EXERCISE

How Ready Are You?

Instructions: Please circle "Yes," "No," or "Undecided" below each statement.

1. Getting healthy is not something I should do or something I need to do. Instead, it's something I *want* to do.

    YES   UNDECIDED   NO

2. I believe diets, pills, and weight-loss gadgets are quick-fix approaches that won't give me the long-term results I want.

    YES   UNDECIDED   NO

3. I am ready to look internally to solve my weight and body-image issues.

    YES   UNDECIDED   NO

4. I value my health and quality of life.

    YES   UNDECIDED   NO

5. I am willing to make taking care of myself a priority in my life.

    YES   UNDECIDED   NO

6. I am ready to exercise and eat healthfully for life-long weight loss and health.

   YES   UNDECIDED   NO

7. I am willing to educate myself about exercise and nutrition.

   YES   UNDECIDED   NO

8. I am ready to take an honest look at my attitudes, thoughts, and behaviors, so I can change what isn't working.

   YES   UNDECIDED   NO

9. I am willing to try new things, even if I feel uncomfortable or self-conscious at first.

   YES   UNDECIDED   NO

10. I am willing to take the time necessary to be successful.

    YES   UNDECIDED   NO

11. I will keep promises to myself.

    YES   UNDECIDED   NO

12. I will reach out to family and friends for support, telling each specifically what I need from her or him.

    YES   UNDECIDED   NO

13. I have faith the decisions I make are the ones that are best for me, regardless of what others think.

    YES   UNDECIDED   NO

14. I believe I can lose weight on my own, without diet books, foods, and pills.

    YES   UNDECIDED   NO

15. I am worth the effort.

    YES   UNDECIDED   NO

How'd you do? The more "Yes" responses you have, the more prepared you are to create your own fitness plan and stick to it. Does that mean you can't do it if you answered "No" to a few? Only you can answer that question. Perhaps it's time you really thought about why you want to lose weight. You're setting yourself up for failure if you don't understand the realities of losing weight and keeping it off for a lifetime.

What You Need to Know About Diets

If you're questioning whether this process will work for you, here's some information to help you decide:

The Great American Pastime: Dieting

The diet industry makes $40 billion a year. Yet the number of obese and overweight individuals continues to grow each year. The U.S. has more dieters, diet books, diet food, and diet centers than any other country on the planet, yet we are the fattest nation. The International Food Information Council estimates that there are currently more than 54 million Americans on a diet who are not getting any thinner. The more we diet, the fatter we get. Research shows that anywhere from 85 to 98 percent of dieters gain their initial weight loss back and many end up heavier than they were before they started dieting.

Definition of a Diet

For the purposes of this book, the word diet refers to a specific plan or program that promises quick weight loss, limits food selections, and usually doesn't say much about changing your eating habits permanently or how critical exercise is to long-term success.

Most diets tell you what you want to hear and leave out what you don't. A few, such as the Atkins Diet® or the South

Beach Diet™, take sound nutritional research to extremes to give you the quick weight-loss results they hope will keep you hooked.

In doing my research, I came across three types of diets:

1. Fad diets—These are the diets that are so unrealistic and restrictive (e.g., cabbage soup, grapefruit), there's no hope of anyone achieving long-term weight loss and maintenance. I suspect many creators of these diets were in it only for the money. I can't imagine anyone creating such a diet to contribute to the health and well-being of its followers.

2. "Just follow me" diets and programs—These are diets (and exercise programs) that someone else has created and is either arrogant or ignorant enough to believe that if it worked for him, it will work for you, too (assuming you follow it exactly).

   These "Just follow me" programs may be created as a result of years of learning and research. Many are created out of a true caring about people's health and wellness. The arrogance enters the picture when it is assumed that all will benefit from that exact approach. Applying the "If it worked for me, it will work for you" premise doesn't work in every situation, as I can attest.

   The Body-for-LIFE® Program created by Bill Phillips was the closest I ever got to trying a diet. I have to admit, the possibility of winning money for losing weight was attractive, although not the best reason to change my eating and exercise habits. I read the book in a matter of hours and was excited to get started. I ignored the uncomfortable feeling I had when I read there an "authorized" list of foods from which I was to eat six days a week, and a "free" day on which I could eat anything I wanted. I started working out as specified in the book, implemented eating five times a day, and planned my meals and workouts ahead of time. I even wrote down what I ate and what I did to exercise.

I soon found myself doing more aerobic exercise and less strength training than what the book said to do. I started eating before I'd exercise in the morning, as I would get so hungry, I'd end up with headaches and stomach cramps. I never did stick to the list of authorized foods. I also became obsessed with food. I was preoccupied with planning every meal and looked forward to my one day off each week, eagerly anticipating all the junk food I would eat that day.

Mr. Phillips may argue I never really gave the program a chance. I would argue, however, that my extreme focus on food and my excitement over gorging on junk food one day a week were anything but healthy.

3. Generalized diets—These diets were created for a specific group of people and then sold to the general population. They are often based upon sound research and serve a purpose when applied on a short-term basis to the population for which they were created. When applied to the general population, however, they can be extreme, restrictive, and even unhealthy.

The South Beach Diet™ is just such an example. Dr. Arthur Agatston created it for his heart patients, who were at risk of heart attack, stroke, or other diseases related to being overweight. His patients had an urgent health-related reason to lose weight.

Why, then, does such a diet get shared with the general population? Dr. Agatston relates in his book that people saw the results and started asking about the diet, so much so that he thought it would be helpful to write a book.

Is it really a surprise that people started asking about the diet? In our "I want it now" society, there are some people who will always be interested in the quick fix, who want to lose weight now, despite taking years to pile it on. There will always be people looking for someone else's answer because they don't want to take the time to determine their own. Selling them an answer that may work for a short time in certain situations is not appropriate and perpetuates the Diet Mindset.

Why Diets Don't Work

There are many reasons diets don't work in the long run. Here are just a few:

Physical

Over time, there is no way to trick your body. Calorie restrictions that are lower than what your body requires cause your body to believe you are starving. In response, your body will hold on to fat and your metabolism slows, making the problem worse.

Simply put, your metabolism is the rate at which your body burns calories. Your metabolism is fueled by adequate caloric intake and exercise, both aerobic exercise and strength training. Further, your metabolism increases with the amount of muscle your body has. Research indicates that if you are losing more than one or two pounds per week, you are decreasing the amount of muscle and increasing the amount of fat in your body. As the amount of fat increases, you must eat fewer calories to avoid getting fat. This, in turn, lowers your metabolism further, and it becomes harder to lose fat. This occurs even if you are consistently exercising.

By unrealistically restricting calories, you are likely to experience uncontrollable food binges, feel hungry all the time, and put your long-term health in jeopardy. What you will never do is lose weight permanently.

Social

We all love food. From a young age, we learn to associate food with family, friends, good times, and even love. Diets don't address this fact. They place unrealistic restrictions on what you eat, and define success in terms of following those restrictions. When you eat something you're not supposed to (and

> *It's medically and physiologically impossible to lose three pounds of fat from the body in a week, let alone the five pounds some plans advertise.*
>
> —Covert Bailey

you will), you feel as though you're a failure. Diets set you up for failure, given the role food plays in our society.

Individual

Many factors influence the way you think about food— your ethnicity, culture, religious beliefs, education, socioeconomic status, and medical history are just a few. Diets don't take these individual differences into account and never address the individual reasons you're overweight. Diet creators don't know your likes and dislikes, where you grew up, or whether you exercise. Only you know these things. Only you can incorporate them into a plan that makes sense for you.

Psychological

Diets don't account for the fact that we crave what we're told we can't have. Diets take away your choices, telling you what you can and can't eat. They're about deprivation, restriction, and doing what you're told. Eating healthfully, however, is about exploring your options and making decisions that are right for you. It's about making choices you want to make, not simply being told what to do.

Financial

The diet industry is a $40-billion-a-year industry whose profits are fueled by your failure at dieting. Think about it. It is in the industry's best interest to keep you fat. Those in the diet industry wouldn't be making $40 billion each year if what they sold you worked.

What If I Still Have Doubts?

So, you still have doubts that you can do this. Keep reading anyway. Surround yourself with those who support your efforts, read stories of those who have succeeded at breaking free from dieting and unhealthy relationships with food, and behave for now as if you have no doubts.

In researching this book, I asked many dieters if they had ever tried losing fat by exercising and eating healthfully, as opposed to dieting. I received a response from a young woman who was recovering from an eating disorder who said she couldn't eat "right," since she has struggled with eating disorders. I hope you recognize, as I did, that the only reason she can't eat right is because she believes she can't.

Belief that you can achieve your goals is vital to accomplishing anything. If you don't believe you can do it, you will consistently undermine your efforts. This does not mean you can't get going if you don't wholeheartedly believe that you can live a healthy lifestyle and be at peace with your body. What it does mean is you can act as if you believe until you actually do. Just get going; don't let the lack of belief hold you back. There will be more on challenging your doubts and negative thinking in Chapter 2.

> *If you think you can, you can. If you think you can't, you're right.*
> —Mary Kay Ash,
> Mary Kay Cosmetics

Make the Decision

The first step in changing your attitudes, thoughts, and behaviors is making the decision to change. Why not make that decision now? Don't wait any longer. Make the commitment to yourself and your health.

The important thing is this: to be able at any moment to sacrifice what we are for what we could become.

—Charles DuBois

The Decision

I make the decision, here and now, to live a more balanced, accepting, and healthy lifestyle. I will make choices out of respect for my body and long-term health. I will make taking care of myself and my body a priority in my life.

Your Signature _____

Date _____

To register your decision online, go to
www.trustyourselftotransform.com

CHAPTER 2

I Can Do It!

PREPARING FOR SUCCESS

Congratulations on your decision to live a more accepting and healthy lifestyle. Now it's time to take action. Here's how:

Ditch the Diet Mindset

Diets are everywhere. Dieting has become the norm and is often treated as a hobby. We all grow up with images of food, exercise, and beauty. These images shape our attitudes and beliefs, usually for the worse. The dieting industry only serves to perpetuate these unhealthy beliefs—what I call the Diet Mindset.

The Diet Mindset plays off your fears and hatred of being fat and can seriously hinder any chances of living a healthy lifestyle. Even someone who has never been on a diet is not immune to the Diet Mindset. An example includes the women who buy low-carb chips, cookies, and pizza after hearing all the low-carb hype, even though they have never been on a low-carbohydrate diet. While I am definitely not suggesting a low-carbohydrate diet, to simply buy the low-carb version of the same junk food you have always eaten is not a

healthy choice and reflects the Diet Mindset. To be successful in long-term weight loss and health, you must change
your mindset from one of diets and quick fixes to one of health
and quality of life.

The characteristics of the Diet Mindset follow. Each of
these aspects individually can be detrimental to your health,
but when added together, can be particularly harmful.

Are You on a Diet or Not?

Dieting encourages black-and-white or all-or-nothing
thinking. There is no in-between when it comes to dieting.
Foods are either good or bad; you can eat them or you can't.
You're either on a diet or you're not; there is no room for
error. People who "slip up" don't just forgive themselves and
move on. You beat yourself up for eating a "forbidden" food,
ditch the diet, brand yourself a failure, and continue down
the path of eating all the foods you've been told you can't.

This attitude so invades our society that even people who
aren't dieting struggle with it consistently. You've started to
eat more fruits, vegetables, and whole grains. You feel really
good about the changes you've made in your eating. Then,
there's a baby shower at work. You decide to have a piece of
cake, which leads to a cookie and some ice cream. Now, you're
filled with guilt and can't believe you allowed yourself to eat
that much. Certain foods become the enemy, and diets perpetuate your unhealthy relationship with food.

It's OK to want chocolate or potato chips periodically.
Dieting sets you up to binge later. It's part of the Diet
Mindset—restricting now, so you can splurge later. Isn't that
what a "cheat" day is all about? If you don't have diet restrictions, there is no such thing as "cheating."

While there are foods that do your body more harm than
good (despite what the food industry would like you to believe), no one food or type of food is solely to blame for obesity.

Realize this, and there would be no need to binge or have a "cheat" day. When you realize you can eat something if you really want it, the choice becomes yours.

It's All in the Numbers

Dieting becomes a numbers game, a game of quantity as opposed to quality. You count carbs, grams, points, or calories; you know how much you weigh from day to day; and you know your BMR and BMI. You become obsessed with the number of calories you eat and how many calories you burn when you exercise (that is, if you do exercise). While it is a good idea to educate yourself by reading food labels, there is no need to be so rigid. This is not a way to experience life. Educating yourself about proper portion sizes and healthy eating will get you where you need to be.

To Weigh or Not to Weigh?

Dieting encourages an unhealthy dependence on the scale for measuring success or failure, so much so that women often feel as though they've failed when the scale doesn't budge, despite other positive signs of success. Think about it. How many times do you hop on the scale in a week, or even a day, hoping to have lost a pound or two?

The scale can play a part in measuring progress, but it must be only a piece of overall assessment. To rely exclusively on the scale can be frustrating and misleading. For example, just because you're losing weight doesn't mean you're losing fat. You could be losing muscle, the very thing that helps to maintain your fat loss. Or just because the scale doesn't move doesn't mean there aren't other positive consequences of your health habits, such as increased muscle mass, better heart health, and lower cholesterol and blood pressure.

You must pay attention to the whole picture and not minimize your results simply because you're not seeing a numerical weight loss. You are finally treating your body and yourself with the respect you deserve. That, in and of itself, is worth celebrating.

It's a Miracle...You're Fixed

Short-term weight loss, not lifelong health, is the goal with dieting. Once the weight is off, you stop the plan, but then what? Now you've lost weight, and you haven't a clue as to how to maintain the loss. You return to your old eating habits as though you're "fixed" and won't gain weight. It's wishful thinking to believe that being thin now allows you to eat whatever you want whenever you want. Diets and supplements rarely focus on the importance of exercise and never teach you how to eat healthfully. You will gain the weight back if you don't have a long-term focus.

A Way of Life?

The dieting industry has helped to create and perpetuate the myth that dieting, if done properly, can be a way of life. It tries to cover up that a diet is truly a diet by using words like plan or program. When doing research for this book, I asked dieters, many of whom were on the Atkins Diet®, if they'd ever tried to lose weight using exercise and healthy eating, as opposed to dieting. Several responded to say that Atkins is not a diet but a "way of life." Bill Phillips, in his book, *Body-for-LIFE®*, writes, "The Body-for-LIFE® Program is just that—for life. It's not something I do for just a certain amount of time. It's the way I live. And it will be for you as well, by the time the next 12 weeks are over."

Call it what you want; it's still a diet.

What people in the industry don't tell you is that diets, inherently, cannot be a way of life. In many instances, you are not eating enough of what your body needs or wants for it to function well. When you are told what to do or what you can and can't eat, it's a life sentence, not a way of life. Educate yourself and make your own decisions about what you eat.

> *It is good to have an end to journey toward, but it is the journey that matters in the end.*
> —Ursula Leguin

It's Time to Enjoy the Journey

Dieting focuses only on the end result. You want to weigh what you weighed in high school, be a certain size, or have a six-inch waist no matter what it takes. While it's critical to have an end result in mind, to be successful, you must pay equal attention to the journey. Staying fit is a life-long process, so you'd better enjoy it along the way. Pick a variety of foods and activities out of respect for your body. Make the journey enjoyable, and your body will take care of the rest.

Focus on the External

Dieters focus on the fat itself and not the reasons they became fat in the first place. Fat becomes the enemy, and you want to eliminate it. The fear and hatred of fat, not wanting to be fit, is the motivation for dieting. Fat is not the problem; it's a symptom of the problem. The problem is the unhealthy lifestyle you've been leading. The more you try to solve the problem with quick-fix, external approaches, the more the so-called solution contributes to the problem.

> *The way we see the problem is the problem.*
> —Stephen R. Covey

Thin Versus Healthy

Dieting focuses on how you look, as opposed to how you feel or how fit you are. Further, the weight-loss industry perpetuates the myth that equates being thin with being healthy. The truth, in fact, is that extreme focus on being thin can be detrimental to your health. Think about the people who have died taking ephedra or Phen-Fen or those who have eating disorders.

Being thin does not mean you are healthy; it simply means you are thin. Someone can be thin but still have a high body-fat percentage, high cholesterol, or clogged arteries from eating unhealthy food.

When I was younger, my friends used to cover themselves with baby oil, go to tanning salons, and literally fry their skin in an effort to look "healthy." They were equating the image of health with the identity of behaving and living healthfully. Many of us spend billions of dollars on beauty products, weight-loss products, and plastic surgery for the same reason—we are chasing after an image instead of striving to live the true identity. Dieting perpetuates an image. The focus on looks is anything but healthy.

> *More than 3000 young people start smoking each day in the U.S. The main reason females start is to lose weight.*
>
> —Source: National Heart, Lung, and Blood Institute

If Only I Were Thin

Diets encourage the belief that life would be so much better if only you were thin. While setting and achieving fat-loss or fitness goals can positively affect other areas of your life, you must realize there could be areas in your life that need work, regardless of how thin or fit you are. Being thin and looking good do not lead to automatic happiness, despite what commercials and advertisements imply.

Focus on Food

Dieting encourages the belief that food is the key to fat loss. This is not the case. Women do have to learn how to eat healthfully when surrounded by unhealthy choices, but unrealistically restricting certain foods or food groups is not the answer. In order to lose fat and keep it off, you must change the body on a systemic level. Food can never do this; only exercise changes the body in this way. In fact, the focus dieting puts on food creates one of the hardest habits to break when changing your focus from dieting to health.

> *Whatever you put your attention on will grow stronger in your life.*
> —Deepak Chopra

I Want It Now!

Dieting encourages setting unrealistic goals and time frames. Have you noticed that people often ask how long it took you to lose weight, as if the faster you do it, the better it is? This is not a competition. It's better to lose thirty pounds and keep it off for good, regardless of how long the initial weight loss takes, than to lose fifty pounds in three months and gain it back within a year.

Worse yet, the diet industry sets and reinforces the expectation that not only should losing weight be quick and easy,

> *In the long run, exercise is the ultimate cure for obesity.*
> —Covert Bailey

but so should everything supposedly associated with weight loss—health, happiness, and quality of life. This expectation often causes people to give up because it's taking too long.

Technology and the media only reinforce the message that faster is better. What if faster isn't better? What if things really worth having, such as health and quality of life, weren't meant to be quick and easy? What if we're so focused on what we can get now, that we've lost sight of what really matters?

It's time to stop looking for short-cuts and do what it really takes to lose weight and keep it off. To be healthy, you must live healthfully. Looking for shortcuts only leads to failure and frustration.

> *There are no shortcuts to anyplace worth going.*
>
> —Beverly Sills

There's Nothing Like a Little Deprivation

The weight-loss industry has created an environment in which food deprivation and restriction are socially-acceptable behaviors. Not only are they acceptable, but encouraged. The media publicize the latest diet as if it is the answer to obesity. Support groups have popped up everywhere to urge you to stay on your diet, answer questions, and swap recipes and products. The International Information Food Council estimates that there are more than 54 million Americans currently on a diet. Those who aren't on a diet will soon be in the minority.

The sad part is, the deprivation and restriction aren't helping our obesity. If we do nothing to stop the rise in obesity, experts estimate that 95 percent of us will be obese by the year 2040. It's time to stop depriving ourselves and live healthfully.

Dieting Is Anything but Healthy

The diet industry encourages the belief that dieting is healthy and in the best interest of your body, so much so that many people believe dieting is necessary for permanent weight loss and long-term health. Regardless of what your friends and family believe, dieting and eating healthfully are not the same things. In fact, dieting is anything but eating healthfully.

Dieting is about ignorance, will power, fear of food, doing what you're told to do, restriction, self-deprivation, and even starvation. It is not healthy.

A Vicious Cycle

Dieting encourages a "quick fix" mentality. It becomes something you do regularly throughout the year. You live in a cycle of diets, hoping to find the one that works for you. Is swimsuit season approaching? Have a wedding you want to attend? Why not pop some pills or try a liquid diet to lose the weight quickly? Dieting becomes such a habit that it doesn't occur to you that regular exercise and eating healthfully could eliminate the need for last-minute weight loss. Just imagine a time when you never have to worry about fitting into that dress or those shorts you haven't worn since last year. Your weight stays consistent, so there are no surprises. This is possible when you choose a healthy lifestyle over dieting.

One Size Does Not Fit All

Dieting creates a "one-size-fits-all" mentality. You become a follower. You are not empowered to change your health for the better by creating your own plan. You rely on someone else to tell you what to do. You are not considered the expert about your own body. A complete stranger assumes that role instead. You are led to believe that you, too, can be thin if only you follow a particular diet or program, and if only you try hard enough. As time goes on, however, the diet becomes harder to maintain and your weight loss slows. Eventually, your weight loss stops, and you start to gain it back. You have failed again. Regardless of the reason for failure, you don't even consider the fact that the diet is the problem. Instead, you blame yourself. Relying on others to tell you what's right for you strips you of your power. Empower yourself and make the choices that are right for you.

I Was Meant to Be Fat!

The cycle of dieting and self-blame eventually leads you to believe it's impossible to lose weight no matter what you do. You believe you no longer have control over your choices. Fat becomes who you are; there is no other possibility. These beliefs can undermine your ability to live a healthy lifestyle. Further, they can stop you from ever trying to lose weight again, since you believe you're doomed to be fat.

> *It is the diet, not you!*

The "AH-HA!" Moment

It's time to forget about finding some magic potion, pill, or diet that will work overnight. It's time to stop blaming yourself and leave dieting behind. Commit to living a healthy lifestyle today. Most importantly, realize that dieting does not work. Arguments over what to eat and what not to eat keep you from looking at the real issues:

1. We eat too much of everything except healthy food.

2. We exercise far too little.

You must let go of dieting completely and realize your body is unique, requiring a customized fitness plan only you can create. There are no quick fixes to permanent fat loss and healthy living. A mindset of health and quality of life must replace the Diet Mindset. The table on page 25 depicts the characteristics of a Diet Mindset versus those of a Quality-of-Life Mindset.

> *...you can never accomplish a worthy end with unworthy means.*
> —Stephen Covey

Diet Mindset	Health/Quality-of-Life Mindset
Efficiency	Effectiveness
Image	Identity
Symptoms	Root causes
Scarcity/Deprivation	Abundance
Control/Willpower	Empowerment/Choice
Programmed	Programmer/Creator
Someone else as expert	You as expert
Techniques/Tips/Formulas	Principles
Structure	Flexibility/Balance
Depletion of time, energy, and money	Investment in long-term health and quality of life

WRITTEN EXERCISE

Shedding the Diet Mindset

Instructions: Look back to the characteristics of the Diet Mindset. How many of them currently apply to you? List those that apply below in the left-hand column. In the right-hand column, challenge each one, citing why you think the characteristic will hinder your focus on health. See the example below.

Characteristic	Challenge
Example: Quick fix—I thought it would be quick and easy.	It was quick at first, but it didn't last.

Change Your Definition of Success

Success in weight loss is measured by how much weight you've lost and how quickly you've lost it. Long-term results and improved health are not included in the definition of success. I cannot count how many times I've heard people say a diet has worked even though they have gained all the weight back. A great example is an Oprah guest speaking of his recent gastric bypass surgery. In explaining his long history of weight loss and gain, he told Oprah he had tried a liquid diet on which he'd lost over 100 pounds, informing Oprah and millions of viewers looking for an answer to their weight issues that "it worked." All I could think was, "If it had worked, you wouldn't be sitting here on TV right now talking about the gastric bypass surgery you just had." Another example is a woman who lost eight pounds within the first two weeks of starting a popular low-carbohydrate diet. She was sharing this information with several co-workers, one of whom responded, "It really does work!"

If your definition of success is losing eight pounds of water weight in two weeks, then yes, that diet does work. Or, if you define success as losing weight and gaining it all back, then try any diet and you will succeed. If, however, you define success as losing body fat and maintaining the loss while improving your health, fitness, and body image, a diet will never do the trick.

If a plan doesn't allow you to maintain it, it doesn't work. Continuing to make such claims gives false credit to diets and misleads anyone who is trying to live more healthfully. Further, you are branding yourself a failure. You're saying the diet worked, yet you gained the weight back, meaning you failed to keep it off.

It's time to create a new definition of success. This definition looks at several measures:

Health

How many healthy changes have you made in your life? Has your physical health improved? How do you feel about your body? Has your body image improved? Are you more interested in treating your body with respect than doing whatever it takes to be thin? Have you stopped obsessing about food?

Fitness

Are you able to lift more weight or perform more repetitions? Have you been able to exercise longer or has your pace improved?

Maintenance

Is your fitness plan becoming a permanent part of your lifestyle? Are your exercise and eating behaviors something you want to continue? Are your behaviors realistic and flexible? How long have you been able to either lose more body fat or maintain that loss?

The Process

Are you achieving your goals and keeping promises to yourself? Are you enjoying the process as much as, if not more than, the results?

Balance

Are you achieving in other areas of your life? Do you feel as though all areas of your life receive the attention they deserve? Are you incorporating all four dimensions of health into your plan?

Happiness

Are you enjoying your life, regardless of your weight? Are you at peace with food, your body, and yourself? Are you practicing self-acceptance, regardless of your size?

These are the true measures of success, not how much weight you've lost in a week or a month. Real success is measured on a continuum. Each healthy change you make is a step in the right direction. Engaging in extreme behaviors, such as restrictive or overindulgent eating is not healthy. Balance, flexibility, and moderation are the worthy goals.

WRITTEN EXERCISE
Your Success Story

Instructions: Take time now to write your success story. Picture what life is like once you've achieved your goals. How do you feel about your body and yourself? What are people saying to you? How are they treating you? What do you see, feel, and hear? Comment on the measures of success previously mentioned. Are you at peace with your body? How fit are you? What are you now able to do? Write it as though you have already achieved what you want. Use the story as motivation, when necessary. As time progresses, revisit your success story regularly and update when appropriate.

Face Your Fears

For many of you, dieting is all you know. It's the only option you've tried for losing weight. So, while you know dieting hasn't gotten you the results you want, it's still scary trying something new, especially a plan you create yourself. What if you don't get the results you want this time? How much will your life have to change for you to live healthfully? Will your friends and family support your decisions?

The most common fears you'll need to face and work through when striving to live more healthfully are: the fear of failure, the fear of the unknown, and the fear of rejection. All three have kept many women from achieving their fitness goals. Don't allow them to keep you from achieving yours.

> *The key to change…is to let go of fear.*
> —Rosanne Cash

Fear of Failure

People who fail believe in failure. People who succeed see their failures as feedback or results to be evaluated. They are simply experiences that move you one step closer to success. You already know what many don't—that dieting doesn't get you the results you want. It's time to determine what does.

Fear of the Unknown

It amazes me how many women are willing to stay in a miserable situation because they are afraid. People would rather deal with the known, no matter how bad it gets, than conquer their fear of trying something new. What if you change employers and still don't like your job? What if you leave an unfulfilling relationship and can't find someone else? Or what if you go

> *If you do what you've always done, you'll get what you've always gotten.*
> —Unknown

through all this work and still don't live a healthier, better-quality life?

You can continue to play "what if" the rest of your life or you can take action. The only way you'll find the answers is to get moving.

Fear of Rejection

With more than 54 million Americans on a diet and an online support group for just about every weight-loss "plan" out there, you've got an automatic support system full of people just waiting to share recipes, answer questions, and provide support when needed. But what if your plan isn't like everyone else's? What if you aren't on The Atkins Diet® or Body-for-LIFE®? What if all your close friends suffer from the Diet Mindset?

Anytime we try something different, we risk not being accepted by others. You must decide whether your health and well-being are more important than being accepted. It is only when you make choices out of respect for yourself and your body, regardless of what others think, that you find true success.

> *As you look at many people's lives, you see that their suffering is in a way gratifying, for they are comfortable in it. They make their lives a living hell, but a comfortable one.*
>
> —Ram Dass

> *Our greatest challenge is to be ourselves in a world that is trying to be like everyone else.*
>
> —Renee Locks

Focus on What You Can Control

People waste much of their time and energy on things they can't control—their past mistakes, why someone else behaved the way she did, or issues in their environment. People who achieve their goals, on the other hand, work on things they can do something about. They learn from their past mistakes and move forward. They don't worry about circumstances over which they have no control, and they realize the only thing they can truly control is how they respond to their world.

The same is true for anyone trying to lose weight and live more healthfully. There is no denying there are many factors that have contributed to your weight and body image, many of which are out of your control. But why focus on those things? Why focus on your family history of obesity or the fact that there's a fast-food restaurant on every corner? That only serves to keep you where you are. Stop fooling yourself. It's time to take responsibility for the decisions that are within your control.

> *Successful people are different; they don't follow the crowd, and those who don't follow the crowd are often criticized for being different.*
>
> —Thomas J. Stanley, Ph.D.

Determine the Real Reasons You're Overweight

Why are you overweight? The simple answer is that you eat too much and move too little. It's time to look deeper, while focusing on the behaviors you can change. You can never lose weight and maintain the loss until you know what caused your weight gain in the first place. You have to know what behavior is not getting you the results you want in order to change it. Do you eat fast food all the time because you have a hectic schedule and hate to cook? Are all your family and friend get-togethers about food? Do you use food to try to fulfill a non-food need? How about exercise? Have you made it a consistent part of your life? Why or why not? You have to acknowledge what you are (or aren't) doing to change your habits.

WRITTEN EXERCISE

Why Are You Really Overweight?

Instructions: List every behavior that is contributing to your being
overweight in the left-hand column. In the right-hand column, list
alternative, healthy behaviors. Get creative and list as many alternative behaviors as you can. Examples are included below:

Current Behavior	Changed Behavior
Example: I don't get enough exercise.	Take the stairs at work. Walk with my husband.
I eat fast food on the way home from work because I'm starving.	Have healthy food in my car. Eat a healthy snack mid- afternoon, so I'm not hungry when driving home. Take a different route home, so I'm not tempted by fast-food restaurants.

Broaden Your Definition of Health

When most people think of health as it relates to losing weight, they think only about physical health. There are, however, several dimensions of health that all must be addressed for weight loss and lifelong health to occur.

While different words have been used to describe the dimensions of health, most philosophies agree that there are four: physical, mental, spiritual, and social. You must nurture each dimension to be most effective. When you encourage any one area, the others benefit. When you neglect one, all suffer.

Physical	*Mental*
• Caring for your physical body through exercise, nutrition, sleep, and stress management	• Learning • Reading • Planning
Spiritual	*Social*
• Clarifying and living your values • Meditation • Prayer	• Relationships • Support • Empathy • Helping Others

I like to think of it in terms of energy. When each area of your life is in balance, you feel energized. There is a synergy, and you feel as though everything is coming together. This synergy creates even more energy. Whereas, when one or more areas are out of sync, it drains energy from all the others.

As in any aspect of life, you must address each dimension of health in an appropriate and balanced manner for optimal effectiveness of your fitness plan. Each person will approach each dimension differently. Below are examples of how each dimension may be included in your plan:

Physical	*Mental*
• Aerobic exercise • Strength training • Relaxation/rest • Sleep • Stretching • Stress management	• Educating yourself on health and nutrition • Creating your plan • Problem solving through obstacles • Using visualization to achieve goals
Spiritual	*Social*
• Meditation • Prayer • Communing with nature • Listening to uplifting music • Setting goals in accordance with what you value	• Forming a support network • Connecting with others who have struggled with their weight or body image • Providing support and empathy to others

Stop Saboteurs

Leaving diets and the Diet Mindset behind can be difficult. Anticipating your saboteurs helps prepare for this inevitability.

The Saboteur You Least Expect

The worst saboteur on your journey to health may be you. Your negative attitudes, beliefs, and internal dialogue can do more to damage your capabilities than anyone externally. Perhaps you don't believe you can do it. You're afraid you'll fail again, so why even try?

For whatever reason, you find yourself making poor choices, choices that hinder your progress. Look at whether you're being too hard on yourself. Remember the point is to eliminate the rules and restrictions of dieting. Are you eating your favorite not-so-healthy foods periodically and in moderation, or is it becoming a consistent pattern? If you see a pattern of poor choices developing, it's time to think about why.

I Just Can't Do This!

Every single one of us has experienced negative self-talk at some point in our lives. We may put ourselves down or say we can't do something. Have you ever thought about the impact this self-talk has on your behavior and your self-esteem? Are you going to put your utmost effort into something you keep telling yourself you can't achieve? Would you allow someone else to tell you you're ugly or lazy or not worth the effort? Then why do you allow yourself to do it?

The first step in eliminating any behavior is acknowledging that it exists and that it's something you want to eliminate.

> *We are what we think. All that we are arises with our thoughts. With our thoughts, we make our world.*
>
> —Buddha

WRITTEN EXERCISE

Eliminating Your Negative Self-Talk

Instructions: For the next week, write down anything negative you tell yourself internally. The goal is to get an idea of what negative messages you consistently give yourself. Once that's complete, challenge the validity of each message using the table below. Examples have been included.

Internal Dialogue	Challenge
Example: I can't do this.	I have made the decision to do this, and I will follow through.
I will always be fat.	Being fat is a choice; I can also choose to be thin.

Your responsibility going forward is to challenge the validity of each negative message, substituting it with a positive one. This allows you to acknowledge the positive changes you're making in your life and to build upon them.

Stop the Comparison

Comparisons of people are made every day in school, in sports, on the job, and even in our families. Decisions are made based upon these comparisons—who's smarter, faster, better? We're taught there's a winner and a loser, and that it's better to be the winner.

There is no room for comparison when striving to live a healthy lifestyle. Someone is always going to be thinner or more muscular than you are. There is always going to be someone who has lost weight more quickly, works out more, can lift more weight, or eats more healthfully than you do. Comparing yourself and your situation to others' only inflates or diminishes your achievements. It creates animosity and a competitive environment that hinder your progress. Comparison with others also allows you to defend your excuses for not doing all you can to live healthfully. "She's younger, so it's easier for her to lose weight." "She doesn't have as much weight to lose as I do." "She doesn't have as long a commute as I do, so she has the time to work out." "She has no idea how tiring it is having two children at home." The list goes on and on. You have to recognize these comparisons for what they are—excuses. Yes, they may be legitimate reasons why living a healthy lifestyle is difficult for you. But you must stop focusing on the problems and focus on the solutions to achieve what you want to achieve. Obsessing about the problems keeps you stuck; you become incapable of seeing solutions when you're focused so much on the problems.

Progress is relative and individual. A supportive, cooperative environment is best for achieving permanent weight loss and gain of health and better quality of life. Comparison and competition destroy such an environment.

Oh, the Guilt!

Many of you believe you need to put everyone else's needs before your own, and, if you don't, you're being selfish. Wipe that thought out of your minds right now. Taking care of yourself is, in fact, the most unselfish thing you can do. (Yes, I said unselfish.) You cannot take care of others well until you take care of yourself. Remember this always.

Your Environment

We live in an environment that promotes too much eating and too little activity. Kelly D. Brownell in his book *Food Fight*, says, "We are literally eating ourselves to death." Yet we have all ignored the obesity crisis until recently, believing the overweight and obese are either weak or lazy, and deserve to be fat.

Now, almost two-thirds of American adults are either overweight or obese. If this trend continues unchecked, experts say 95 percent of us will be obese by the year 2040. Our children are gaining weight so quickly that they are now getting diseases that were once only associated with adults, such as type II diabetes. We must stop ignoring the problem and take responsibility for the choices we make in response to our environment.

While our environment rarely encourages healthful decisions, we each can decide how our surroundings will affect us. Will you continue to allow yourself to be a victim of your circumstances? Or will you choose a different response? The freedom to choose your

> Anytime we think the problem is "out there," that thought is the problem. We disempower ourselves.
> —Stephen R. Covey

response, regardless of the environment, is your greatest power. Use it wisely.

Your Community

Suburban sprawl; lack of sidewalks and trails; busy, unsafe streets; and worsening air pollution all discourage outdoor activity. Unless you live in a home built before 1974, your community is likely to be what I call a "pop-up" community. These are the communities in which developers find a piece of land in the middle of nowhere and build homes. These communities rarely have sidewalks and, if they do, they typically don't extend beyond the community itself. You have to drive everywhere you go, as busy roadways with no shoulders for walking or biking often surround these neighborhoods. Gone are the days you could walk to the grocery store or to a restaurant. Instead, you have to make it a point to walk purely for the sake of exercise.

The Food You Eat

Unhealthy food is everywhere you look. It's convenient, fast, cheap, and produced with fat, sugar, and flavors to keep you coming back for more. Worse yet, portion sizes are expanding everywhere—restaurants, vending machines, convenience stores, supermarkets, and even at home. This is true to the extent that we've lost sight of what an appropriate portion size is. Couple the portion-size increase with the fact that 67 percent of Americans report eating whatever is on their plates, regardless of how much food is there, and it spells disaster for your health and for your waistline.

> *The average woman eats 335 more calories a day than she did in the 1970s.*
>
> —Source: *Oxygen Magazine*, June 2004

Technology

The inventions of modern-day society, such as escalators, moving walkways, elevators, computers, the Internet, and e-mail have eliminated the need for physical activity. You literally have to make a conscious decision to exercise. Further, technology encourages the belief that all things should be quick and easy, and the quicker and easier they are, the better. This belief, no matter how much you'd like it to be true, does not apply to living a healthy lifestyle. Making the changes necessary to live healthfully is not quick and, for many, is not easy.

Big Industry

Besides the diet industry, there are two other forces working hard to keep you fat and confused: the media and food industries.

The Media

The latest diet, the obesity crisis, and weight-loss research have become hot topics in the media lately. In fact, many people consider the media a major (if not their only) source for health and nutrition information, believing they'll receive reliable, unbiased information. Basic nutrition information has remained the same for over fifty years, yet the media require "news." They want breakthroughs and controversy, which often makes the information they report incomplete, contradictory, and confusing. Further, much of the media get their information from food industry representatives, the very people who have a vested interest in having you eat more food.

The Food Industry

The food industry's job is to sell you food. The more food they can get you to buy, the more money in their pockets and in those of their shareholders. The food industry will do anything it can to create an environment that supports an "Eat more" message. Not only do they produce enough food to provide every woman, man, and child in the United States with 3,800 calories (almost double what the average adult needs), but they spend billions of dollars each year learning what tempts us most. Then they allocate nearly 70 percent of the $33 billion they spend on advertising each year pushing their most unhealthy products—soft drinks, convenience foods, candy, desserts, snacks, and alcohol. However, they spend just over two percent of their marketing budget advertising beans, whole grains, fruits, and vegetables.

Furthermore, the industry will use any tactic to get you to buy their products. They:

- Manipulate their food by adding vitamins and minerals or decreasing fat in an effort to get you to believe their most processed products are healthy.

- Slap claims on their packaging such as "high in fiber" or "lowers cholesterol" to get you to perceive their products as healthy, or at least more healthy than their competitors'.

- Use research and science to confuse the public and hide how much harm unhealthy foods can do to our bodies.

- Market their most unhealthy products specifically to children, minorities, and the poor to expand their customer base.

- Oppose food labels and nutrition information that would educate consumers about what they're eating.

- Design new, unhealthy, and unnecessary products every year to grab business away from competitors.

- Increase portion size, while keeping costs low, so consumers eat more.

- Perpetuate the myth that all foods (including their most high-calorie, high-fat, high-sugar products) can be included in a healthy eating plan.

What the food industry will never do is tell you what you need to eat to live healthfully, as the foods that are the unhealthiest for you are the foods that make them the most money.

Other People
No Comments, Please

Everyone has something to say about weight loss. The diet industry has created a Diet Mindset society. While

> *Food companies will make and market any product that sells, regardless of its nutritional value or its effect on health.*
> —Marion Nestle,
> *Food Politics*

some ideas can be helpful, remember that health, not just weight loss, is your ultimate goal. Many may question what you're doing, give advice, or even give you attitude. If you're sure the comments aren't out of a legitimate concern about your plan, do your best to ignore them. Stick to what works for you and don't let others allow you to doubt yourself.

Your Friends and Family

When you make a change in your life, those closest to you are affected by that change. They may fear you'll grow apart from them or sit in judgment of their extra weight. Perhaps they fear losing a close friend or a loved spouse. It is important you reach out to these people early on. Tell your friends and family how important your plan is to you, what you think will change, how important their relationships are to you, and ask for their support, telling them what you need from them.

Despite your trying to involve them, there could be people in your life who feel threatened by the changes you're making. Realize that this will happen and be prepared for it. Keep the lines of communication open and listen to what they have to say initially, keeping an ear out for any legitimate concerns they may have. Truly seek to understand their reservations, so you can best address them. Use this as an opportunity to strengthen your closest relationships, while limiting time with people who continue to be unsupportive or intolerant of the changes you're making.

Fighting Back

Our environment is designed to encourage us to eat more and move as little as possible. Powerful industries spend billions of dollars to manipulate your thoughts and actions. Expert advertising, brilliant images, and skillful sounds program you to eat more, believe diets are the key to weight loss, expect weight loss to be quick and easy, and accept that you cannot lose weight on your own.

It's time to stop being manipulated and start directing your life. Make decisions based upon your goals and values, not the messages the diet, advertising, and food industries send your way. You can be lured by junk food or you can make the decision to eat healthfully out of respect for your body. You can continue to try diet after diet or do what it takes to lose weight and keep it off. Despite the powerful, unhealthy forces surrounding you, you can choose your responses. Choose the actions that get you what you want.

Create a Comprehensive Support System

One of the most commonly suggested ways for you to stay motivated is to build a comprehensive support system in which being overweight and unfit is not an option. The more people you have around you living a healthy lifestyle, the easier it is for you to maintain your lifestyle and the thicker the barrier between you and the unhealthy messages that bombard you every day.

When creating a support network, there are two types of people you want to include:

- *Those who are in it with you.* These are the people who have similar goals to yours. They have weight to lose and know exercising and eating healthfully are the way to lose it. This group could include an overweight friend, your family members, or someone you meet online.

- *Those who already live a fit lifestyle and have done so for some time.* These people may have once been overweight and decided to make a change or have always recognized the value of living healthfully. They enjoy fitness and are committed to living a healthy lifestyle. These people often include fitness professionals, such as personal trainers, nutritionists, and coaches. These are the people to lean on when all you want to do is sit on the couch and eat junk food.

> *Keep away from the people who try and belittle your ambitions. Small people always do that, but the really great make you feel that you, too, can become great.*
> —Mark Twain

When choosing the members of your support system, choose carefully. You want people who will be supportive of the decisions you make, even if their choices are different. Look for people who are positive and who will hold you accountable.

While having supportive people around you helps achieve any goal, the reality is that not everyone you know will realize the importance of fitness. In fact, some people are neither supportive nor tolerant of those living healthfully. While you want to surround yourself with as many supportive people as possible, your resolve and persistence in achieving your goals is what matters most. You must make the decisions that are right for you, regardless of what others do, say, or think.

Creating Your Support Network

The more people you have surrounding you who live a healthy lifestyle, the less likely you are to go back to your old exercise and eating habits. Let's take a look at your current support system, as well as what help you'd like to add.

Your Current Support Network

Instructions: List all the current people in your life who you think could be part of your support network as your relationships stand. These are people who understand what you'll be going through and who can provide intelligent support.

WRITTEN EXERCISES
Creating Your Support Network

Your Ideal Support Network

Instructions: Now, list the supports you would like to have in your life. Maybe you aren't good friends with many of your neighbors. Is it time to start reaching out? Or, perhaps, you've always wanted to try a session with a personal trainer or nutritionist. Now's the time! List below anyone and everyone you think could help you on your journey to health. Add these steps to your plan.

WRITTEN EXERCISE

How Will Your Journey to Health Affect Those Closest to You?

Instructions: Your journey will have an impact on others in your life. It's time to consider all the ways it may affect your family and friends. Write down everything you can think of, even the smallest changes. Include everything from how the food in the house will change to how your friends could feel left behind as you start incorporating healthy changes into your life.

Once complete, talk to those who you feel will be most affected. Include this as a step in your plan. This will help derail possible conflicts and stabilize your current support network.

Make You Your Priority

Diets take you, as an individual, out of the equation. They are plans rolled out to the general public, as if each person is like everyone else. It's time to focus only on you. You must be your first priority when creating your own plan. You have a different culture, ethnicity, family history, goal set, and definition of health. It is necessary to be aware of those differences and account for them in any long-term plan you set for yourself.

Only you can determine the best way to fit fitness into your life. A customized fitness plan can help you determine realistic goals, conquer obstacles, and shed the Diet Mindset forever.

Educate Yourself

Any time you want to change the results you're getting, you have to change your behavior.

In order to change your behavior, you have to know enough about yourself to determine what behavior is change-worthy. Written exercises have been included throughout the book to help you learn more about yourself and your current behavior. You must also possess enough information about exercise and nutrition to adopt the behaviors that will get you the results you want.

> *Futility is doing the same thing over and over and expecting different results.*
> —Nicholas Boothman

Educate Yourself is broken into two parts to teach you what you need to know to make the decisions that are best for you.

The first section is *Exercise Basics* and includes information on both aerobic exercise and strength training. The second section, called *Eating Well*, provides the nutrition basics that will get you started eating more healthfully.

> *Self-education is, I firmly believe, the only kind of education there is.*
>
> —Isaac Asimov

Exercise Basics

Aerobic Exercise

What Does Aerobic Mean?

Aerobic exercise is any repetitive activity that uses oxygen for energy and is challenging enough to increase your heart rate. Covert Bailey, in his book, *Smart Exercise*, defines aerobic as anything: a) using the large muscles of the lower body, b) creating heavy breathing, and c) lasting at least twelve to fifteen minutes in length without interruption. Examples of aerobic activity include:

- Biking
- Hiking
- Jumping rope
- Swimming
- Dancing
- Rowing
- Fast-paced walking

The Benefits of Aerobic Exercise

There are many benefits of aerobic exercise. Regular exercise can:

- Strengthen your heart
- Increase your energy levels while providing resistance to fatigue
- Increase endurance
- Decrease tension, depression, and anxiety
- Improve mood
- Help you sleep better
- Make your heart more efficient, so it pumps more blood with fewer beats

- Make your lungs more efficient, so they process more oxygen with less effort
- Improve self-esteem
- Help you lose weight and maintain that loss
- Improve your body's ability to deliver oxygen to working muscles
- Lower and help control blood pressure
- Reduce your total cholesterol, increasing HDL (good cholesterol), while decreasing LDL (bad cholesterol)
- Reduce your risk of heart disease, type II diabetes, certain cancers (colon and breast), and stroke
- Improve your immune system
- Improve your quality of life

Strategies for Success
Aerobic Warm Up

As you warm up, the temperature inside your muscles actually warms up, as well. This allows your body to use oxygen more efficiently and makes your muscles more pliable and less susceptible to injury. When you don't warm up, your body lacks the oxygen it needs to work out aerobically. Therefore, you work without using oxygen, tire more quickly, and burn less fat overall.

All that's necessary to warm up is five to fifteen minutes of aerobic exercise at an easy pace. It can be a different exercise from what you'll do eventually, or it can be a slower version of the forthcoming activity. When warming up, you should be breathing harder than when you're not exercising but not as hard as during your actual workout. The longer you intend to work out and the more out of shape you are, the longer your warm up should be.

A survey conducted by Consumers Union of more than 32,000 people found that 83 percent of those who dropped an average of thirty-seven pounds and kept it off for a minimum of five years exercised aerobically at least three times a week, calling it their number one weight-control strategy.

Aerobic Cool Down

The purpose of cooling down is the opposite of warming up. You want to ease out of whatever you're doing by making incremental decreases in speed so your body temperature returns to normal. This decreases the chance of nausea, dizziness, fainting, and undue stress on your heart. Cooling down should last five to fifteen minutes, depending upon how hard you exercised.

Scheduling Your Workouts

Schedule your workout as you would a meeting at work or an outing with your kids. It must become as important as brushing your teeth, picking the kids up from school, or going to the office.

Mix It Up

The best way to achieve effective results is to vary your workouts. At a minimum, you want to change your workout every three to six weeks to ensure your body stays challenged. Ways to vary your aerobic routine include changing the:

- Frequency—You can differ how many times you work out in a day or week. For example, if you are currently walking two times a week, add another session when you're ready. For those of you who have limited amounts of time during the day, you can work out for twenty minutes in the morning and twenty minutes in the afternoon or evening.

- Duration—You can also increase the length of time you exercise. Challenge yourself to extend the period of your aerobic sessions. If you began walking for twenty minutes a day, after three or four weeks, try twenty-five minutes. Once twenty-five minutes is no longer challenging, try thirty minutes.

- Intensity—Intensity refers to how hard you're exercising. While you want to consistently challenge your body to get the results you want, you can use a lower intensity if you've worked out harder the day before. In general, the higher the intensity, the less time you need to spend exercising. This doesn't mean you want to work out every day at a high intensity, as this can lead to fatigue and injury. But, if you know you've got a full day and would still like to exercise, you can hop on your bike and go for a fifteen-minute high-intensity ride. Or you can try interval training, which refers to alternating higher and lower intensities of exertion. You could go for three minutes at a lower intensity and two minutes of all-out exercise, alternating the two intervals for fifteen to twenty minutes.

- Type of Exercise—You can also vary what you do to get your exercise. If you're tired of walking, you may want to try biking or using a rowing machine. It's a good idea to alternate between at least two types (this can also include strength training, which will be discussed in the next section) of exercise consistently. This keeps your body challenged, is more likely to keep you motivated, and helps prevent injury from doing the same movements over and over.

Overtraining
How Much Is Too Much Exercise?

While it is unlikely a beginning or moderate exerciser will overtrain, it is important to realize that you can do too much exercise with too little rest. The level at which overtraining occurs is different for everyone, so it is important to pay attention to your body and how you feel. Symptoms of overtraining include:

- Irritability
- Trouble sleeping
- Loss of appetite
- Lack of concentration
- Fatigue
- Decrease in strength or fitness despite working harder

How to Avoid Overtraining

Be sure not to: 1. Exercise too much, 2. Eat too little, or 3. Get too little rest. All three of these contribute to overtraining.

EXERCISE

The key with exercise is to alternate longer, less-intense workouts with shorter, more-intense ones. This will ensure you're not consistently exercising too hard or too long.

FOOD

You've got to be sure to feed your body enough calories and nutrients when living an active lifestyle. When switching from a dieting lifestyle to a healthy one, we often start exercising without doing much to change the amount or types of food we eat, figuring we'll lose more weight if we work out more while keeping our caloric intake the same. Remember, this will only throw your body into starvation mode and may contribute to overtraining.

While it's not necessary to change all unhealthy eating habits at once, you must eat enough to support your exercise. This may mean an increase in calories, particularly in whole-grain, unrefined carbohydrates. Fruits, vegetables, and whole-grain breads, pastas, and cereals provide your body the energy it needs to keep moving.

REST

We mistakenly think our fitness grows during exercise when, in fact, it grows during rest periods. Your body needs time off to repair and grow. Back-to-back intense workouts mean your body has no time to repair itself and prepare for your next workout; it is in a constant state of breakdown. Alternating light workouts with more intense ones and periodically taking a day off completely will provide the rest your body needs.

What's Best?

How long should you exercise? How often? When? Which exercise is best? We ask these questions as if there's one answer for everyone. It's our quick-fix, "I want it now" mentality appearing once again. Fitness is not a one-size-fits-all proposition. While I provide information to help address each of these questions, you have to determine what is best for you—what will keep you motivated and moving.

Which Exercise Is Best?

Depending upon what you read, anything from walking to rowing to cross-country skiing is considered the "best" exercise. Regardless of the exercise you choose, the key to success is

> *The best exercise is the one you'll do consistently.*

consistency. Start with any exercise you enjoy, adding new ones as you're ready.

How Long and Often Should I Exercise?

How long and often you work out depends on the intensity of exercise and the type of lifestyle you want to maintain. For beginners, most experts recommend twenty to thirty minutes of aerobic exercise three times a week. As your body adjusts to this level of exercise, you want to increase the frequency, duration, or intensity of exercise you are doing to continue receiving maximum results and benefits.

Initially, don't get too hung up on exercising a certain number of minutes. Do what you can while challenging yourself, striving to increase the amount of activity you get weekly. Keep in mind, the more muscle you use for an exercise, the less you have to do of it to get results. This guideline can help you choose which exercise to do in a given day. If you're short on time, you can choose an exercise that uses more muscle, such as biking, over an activity that uses less muscle, like walking. Or, you can choose to make your walk more demanding by including a few hills or by carrying a back-pack.

Calorie Counting to Determine Length

I've seen people at the gym allowing calorie count to determine the length of their workout. Not only can calorie counters on exercise equipment be incorrect by as much as 50 percent, many calories are burned after your workout is over. Further, counting calories encourages you to stop as soon as the magic number is reached. You see exercise only as a means to burn calories, as opposed to something that can change your body and your health.

How Hard Should I Work Out?

You want to work out hard enough to challenge your body. This is what leads to improved cardiovascular functioning and efficient weight loss. The easiest way to know whether you're challenging yourself is by how you feel. You should be breathing deeply and be able to talk, but not comfortably. Go too slowly, and the intensity isn't great enough to produce the results you want. Go too fast, and you tire quickly, which will not improve your aerobic capacity.

Does this mean that anything besides aerobic exercise at this level of intensity is useless? No. The ultimate goal is to live a fit, active lifestyle. Variety of activity and speed will keep you motivated and your body challenged.

Do What Works for You

When determining all aspects of your workout, you want to be sure to take your schedule and your situation into account. If you work late every Monday night and come home exhausted, it makes no sense to schedule an intense workout session for that evening. Perhaps you want to go for a quick walk, take the day off, or work out in the morning. Do what works for you. That is the only way to succeed.

Strength Training
What Does Anaerobic Mean?

Anaerobic literally means without oxygen. These are activities that require a high-energy output and don't last very long, as the body gets tired quickly. Examples of anaerobic activity include:

- Sprinting
- Strength training
- Golfing
- Calisthenics

Benefits of Strength Training

Regular strength training can:

- Help control/maintain body weight
- Increase muscular strength
- Increase your stamina and ability to do work continuously
- Reshape your body
- Strengthen your bones
- Increase your muscular endurance
- Prevent/lessen injury

> *We know that muscle is responsible for burning up to 90 percent of the calories we eat every day.*
>
> —Covert Bailey

> *By age seventy-four, two-thirds of American women can't lift even ten pounds.*

- Maintain or improve joint integrity
- Help you maintain an independent lifestyle
- Improve your balance and coordination
- Improve your self-esteem—when you look stronger and are stronger, you feel stronger and more capable

The National Osteoporosis Foundation predicts the number of Americans who have osteoporosis to increase to 41 million in the next ten years.

Intimidation Factor

Women often feel intimidated by lifting weights. Here are some strategies for getting over that anxiety:

- Start with machines. This decreases the chance of injury when learning how to lift for the first time. It also decreases the odds of using improper form, although that is still possible. Using machines can build your confidence.
- Hire a personal trainer to teach you proper technique for both machines and free weights.
- Go with a friend who knows what she's doing.
- Buy some free weights and teach yourself at home using books and magazines. There are many wonderfully illustrated resources showing proper technique. See Healthy Resources at the back of this book and at www.trustyour selftotransform.com.

Basic Lifting Lingo

Repetition: Often referred to as a rep, a repetition is one complete exercise movement. For example, to lift a weight straight above your head and then lower it to your shoulder is one repetition of the shoulder press exercise.

Set: A set consists of a group of repetitions that are done consecutively. For example, if you were to do ten repetitions of the shoulder press exercise, that would be considered one set. If you were to rest and do ten more repetitions, that would be two sets.

Concentric action: This is the action in which the muscle is shortening during strength training. For example, a dumbbell being lifted in a biceps curl is considered concentric action.

Eccentric action: This is the action in which the muscle lengthens. During the biceps curl, the eccentric action occurs when the dumbbell is lowered.

Strategies for Success
Strength-Training Warm Up
    To decrease the likelihood of injury, you need to warm up your entire body with at least five minutes of light aerobic exercise. The warm up increases the temperature of your muscles, making them more pliable and more resistant to injury. The heavier the workout you have planned, the longer the warm up needs to be, with a maximum being twelve to fifteen minutes. To warm up the specific muscles being stressed, follow the aerobic warm up with a light set of the exercise you intend to perform.

Build a Solid Foundation
    When starting a strength-training program, you want to build a solid foundation by learning the proper form of every exercise and by building overall muscle strength. The first step is to master form using no to low weight. Slowly add more weight as you become more comfortable with a particular movement. You also want to include all major muscle groups in your workout to ensure increased overall strength and the most effective results. The major muscle groups include your:

- Butt (gluteus maximus or glutes)
- Front thighs (quadriceps or quads)
- Back thighs (hamstrings or hams)
- Calves
- Chest (pectoralis or pecs)
- Back
- Shoulders (deltoids or delts)
- Stomach (rectus abdominus or abs)
- Front upper arm (biceps or bis)
- Back upper arm (triceps or tris)

Challenge Your Muscles

The myth that women will get huge muscles unless they lift light weights still persists. There are two prerequisites for becoming huge: 1. Lifting extremely heavy weights and 2. Having the genetics that will allow for the development of huge muscles. Most women don't meet these conditions. Without challenging your muscles beyond what is normal, you won't be able to change your muscle strength or size. Consistently lifting two- and five-pound weights won't do it. Neither will those health-club classes in which you lift weights sixty-two times in a row. If you can lift a weight that many times, it isn't heavy enough.

How your muscles respond to strength training is determined by genetics, and to get any response, you must challenge the muscle.

> *...the sort of exercise that has the possibility of truly sculpting and reforming the body is a far cry from what most women do.*
>
> —Gina Kolata

Exercise Your Muscles in the Right Order

Exercise larger muscles before smaller ones for the most effective and challenging workout. Working smaller muscles first makes them less effective in helping the large muscles when being exercised and tires the larger adjacent muscles, compromising your workout. To exercise your muscles in the right order, you must know which muscles are larger and which are smaller.

When choosing the sequence of your exercises, it's helpful to think of the body in three segments: upper body, middle body, and lower body. Within each segment, the proper order is listed below, with the largest muscles being listed first. When I use "and/or" it doesn't matter which muscle is exercised first.

Upper	Middle	Lower
Chest and/or back	Abs and/or back	Butt
Shoulders		Thighs
Bis and/or tris		Calves and/or shins
Wrists		

Grab a Spot

A spot means you have someone standing by to help in case you can't lift the weight. You don't need a spotter all the time, but one can be helpful when:

- You're trying a new exercise
- You want to challenge yourself by lifting more weight or doing more repetitions

When using a spot, be sure your spotter knows proper spotting technique, feels confident she can help, and takes her role as a spotter seriously.

Remember to Breathe

When you're not breathing as you exercise, your blood pressure can rise to abnormally high levels, putting your health at risk. Holding your breath for consecutive repetitions can also lead to dizziness and fainting. Previous research has always suggested exhaling during the more strenuous part of the exercise and inhaling during the less strenuous part. More recent research from The American Council on Exercise, however, found that breathing at a relaxed, natural pace is the best way to breathe when lifting weights. Regardless of which technique you choose, the important thing to remember is just to breathe.

Give It a Rest

Your muscles need at least forty-eight hours rest in between workouts. In other words, you never want to exercise the same muscle on consecutive days. When you strength train, your muscle fibers tear. Muscle growth and increases in strength occur during rest, when the muscle repairs itself. If you continue to work the same muscles every day, your muscles become overtrained, and you grow weaker, not stronger. Your muscles need time to rest and repair themselves.

No Pain, No Gain?

If you are new to weight lifting or haven't lifted for a while, muscle soreness is common twenty-four to forty-eight hours after exercise. Don't let it stop you from exercising. It is normal to experience soreness for the first week or two.

For many diehard weight lifters, muscle soreness has been a sought-after sign of an effective workout. This is not the case. If you consistently experience soreness after your workouts, you are either lifting too much weight or using improper form.

Strength-Training Cool Down

Ending your workout with a few minutes of light aerobic activity helps to slow your pulse, blood pressure, and breathing. It has also been shown to minimize after-workout muscle soreness.

Keep It Interesting

The best way to achieve effective results is to vary your workouts. Some women choose to change their workouts every week. At a minimum, you want to change your workout every three to six weeks to ensure your muscles stay challenged. Be sure to master proper form on your old exercises before learning new ones. Ways to vary your workout include changing the:

- Amount of weight used
- Number of reps per set
- Number of sets per muscle
- Amount of rest between sets
- Type of resistance used (e.g., machines, free weights, bands, your own body weight)
- Number of exercises used for each muscle group
- Order of the exercises for each muscle group
- Speed of performing the exercise

What's Best?

Machines Versus Free Weights

There are advantages and disadvantages to using both machines and free weights (see below). Start with whatever makes sense for you. You may exercise at home and don't want to buy expensive weight machines, or you may have a club membership with access to both but feel more comfortable starting with machines. You may enjoy doing certain exercises on machines and others with free weights. It's up to you. This is your plan. While using different types of resistance offers the variety your body needs, you want to do whatever you enjoy most, so you're more likely to stick with it.

FREE WEIGHTS

Advantages:

- Your body uses the help of surrounding muscles to lift them, thus developing greater overall strength.

- You can exercise just about every muscle in the body with free weights, whereas machines typically do one or two exercises each.
- You can also modify an exercise if you have an injury or limited range of motion.
- Free-weight exercises more closely resemble natural body movements.
- For those interested in having a home gym, free weights are less expensive and take up less space.

Disadvantages:

- Training alone can be more dangerous. You must be sure to use proper form and not lift too much weight.
- It is time-consuming to change the weight on a dumbbell or barbell.
- You often cannot achieve isolation of a muscle or muscle group.

MACHINES
Advantages:

- They can be safer, as you're less likely to lose control while on a machine. However, it is still possible to injure yourself by lifting too much weight.
- Using machines increases the likelihood of using proper form, since machines have less freedom of motion than free weights. Using machines, however, does not guarantee good form.
- They are easy to use and efficient—most machines require you to move a pin to adjust the weight, as opposed to adding and removing weight plates from a dumbbell or barbell. This can make it much easier to squeeze in a workout any time of day.

- Instead of exercising other muscles, you can isolate a particular muscle. This can be helpful if you need to develop a particular muscle for sports or due to weakness.

Disadvantages:

- Women, especially those who are very tall or very short, may find it difficult to use machines, as they are built with the average-sized man in mind.

- Machines often don't provide the freedom of movement necessary for those with injuries or limited range of movement.

- As you progress, machines may not provide enough muscle development or speed for sport-specific training.

The "Right" Number of Reps

There are several opinions about how many repetitions a woman should perform in each set. Some say women should only do high numbers of reps to avoid "bulking up." Some say the right number is eight to twelve repetitions. Others say the number of reps should depend upon your goal, doing fewer reps with more weight for larger, stronger muscles and higher reps with low weight to improve fitness. What these answers don't take into account is individual differences in response to strength training. For example, your body may respond quickly to lifting minimal weight, or you may have to lift heavy weights to get any response. Keep in mind that different body parts respond differently to training. Your legs may need heavy weights to respond, whereas your shoulders respond to minimal weight. Once you've mastered form, experiment to see what your body best responds to.

How Many Sets?

When first starting out, try one set, focusing on form. As you feel more comfortable, add more sets. Depending upon your goals and your body's response to training, you can do several sets for each muscle group, performing a variety of exercises for each muscle.

Some suggest that performing one set of an exercise for each muscle group is enough to gets results, as long as the one set is performed to failure, meaning it is physically impossible for you to lift more weight using proper form, because you have exhausted the muscle. Most research in this area suggests that beginners may see results from this type of training. But, as the body gets used to training, more is needed to get and keep results. Periodically using one-set training for variety or if you're short on time can be useful, but you want to be careful about working out to failure, as it may encourage injury.

How Frequently Should I Work Each Muscle?

Here again, the research varies, saying anywhere from one to three times per week is effective. In many resources on weight training, the magic number seems to be twice per week. See what works for you. Just remember not to work the same muscle group on consecutive days.

How Fast Should I Perform Reps?

The key word here is variety. Most research suggests that it's effective to take anywhere from one to four seconds for both concentric and eccentric movements. Be sure when performing your reps quickly that you're relying on your muscles and not momentum to do the work.

More Lifting Lingo

Hypertrophy—An increase in muscle size. Hypertrophy does not necessarily indicate an increase in strength, as well.

Periodization—To break down your routine into separate periods. Periods often last anywhere from three to six weeks. Some people use the periods as the point at which they change their routines, even though their overall objectives stay the same. For example, you do the same routine for the first three-week period, then change your workout every three weeks, even though your objective is still to build overall muscle strength and increase fitness. Others may vary their routines frequently throughout the period, while using the change in period to signify a change in objective. For example, the first four-week period is used to increase overall strength, and the next four-week period is used to maintain overall strength while also increasing strength in specific muscles. This approach is often used for preparing for a particular sporting event or season.

Split Routine—Means to split your full-body routine into shorter ones. Two common split routines are to work your upper body one day and your lower body the next, or to perform pulling movements one day and pushing the next. A split routine works well when you:
- Are short on time
- Are tired of doing a full-body routine
- Enjoy focusing on a few muscle groups at once
- Don't have patience for a full-body routine

Upper Body/Lower Body Split Routine
Sample #1

Day of the week	Upper body, lower body, rest
Monday	Upper body and abs
Tuesday	Lower body
Wednesday	Rest
Thursday	Upper body and abs
Friday	Lower body
Saturday	Rest
Sunday	Rest

Sample #2

Day of the week	Upper body, lower body, rest
Monday	Upper body and abs
Tuesday	Rest
Wednesday	Lower body
Thursday	Rest
Friday	Upper body and abs
Saturday	Rest
Sunday	Lower body

Push/Pull Split Routine—This routine separates your pulling muscles (back and bis) from your pushing muscles (chest and tris). When you do your lower body, shoulders, and abs is up to you.

Sample #1

Day of the week	Muscle groups or rest
Monday	Back and bis
Tuesday	Lower body, shoulders, abs
Wednesday	Chest and tris
Thursday	Rest
Friday	Back and bis
Saturday	Lower back, shoulders, abs
Sunday	Chest and tris

Sample #2

Day of the week	Muscle group or rest
Monday	Back, bis, and shoulders
Tuesday	Chest, tris, lower body, abs
Wednesday	Rest
Thursday	Back, bis, and shoulders
Friday	Chest, tris, lower body, abs
Saturday	Rest
Sunday	Rest

You don't need to stick to the day-by-day structure of the samples above. Do what works for you. Some people have busy weekends and prefer not to lift weights on the weekend. Others have more time on weekends. Just be sure not to work the same muscle on consecutive days. Feel free to vary your routine from week to week as your schedule changes.

Advanced Lifting Techniques

Once you've become comfortable with weight lifting and have built a solid foundation while mastering proper form, you may want to try these techniques:

Supersetting—This refers to exercising two anatomically antagonistic (e.g., back and chest, bis and tris, hams and quads) muscles consecutively without rest between the two exercises. You do want to rest briefly between supersets.

Compound sets—These are also often referred to as same-muscle supersets. Here, you alternate two exercises for the same muscle. You rest once you complete both exercises.

Pyramid training—You perform several sets of the same exercise, increasing the weight for each set while decreasing the number of reps.

Sample Pyramid Routine for Biceps

Amount of Weight	Number of Reps
10 lbs.	12
12 lbs.	10
15 lbs.	8
20 lbs	5

Breakdown routine—You lift a heavy weight for as many repetitions as you can while keeping proper form. Then, using a lighter weight, do as many reps as you can, again using proper form.

Eating Well

The Importance of Eating Healthfully

Food habits are often the hardest habits for people to change, especially for those suffering from a Diet Mindset. You may need to re-educate yourself as to what is truly healthy for your body, versus listening to what the latest diets claim to be healthy.

Food is an emotionally charged subject, one about which everyone has something to say. Because everyone has an opinion about food, and because most people don't eat healthfully, it may be difficult to find people who are supportive of your lifestyle. Eating well may also affect your relationships with family and friends, especially if your interactions usually involve food. Add to this the amount of incorrect, confusing, and contradictory information there is out there about food and nutrition, and it can be overwhelming to even consider changing your eating habits. However, adopting healthy eating habits is critical to your long-term success, as what you eat can literally undo your efforts to lose weight and live a healthy lifestyle.

The Three Main Nutrients
Carbohydrates

Carbohydrates include sugars, starches, and certain types of fiber. Most foods contain carbohydrates. Glucose, the simplest carbohydrate, is a necessary fuel for the brain and the body's preferred source of energy. A dominant sugar in food is sucrose, which includes white and brown sugars and table honey. Other sugars include fructose, found in fruits and vegetables, and lactose, found in milk. Starch is found in breads, cereals, beans, pasta, and potatoes. And the best sources of fiber include fruits, vegetables, legumes, and whole-grain foods.

Carbohydrates are easy to blame for the obesity epidemic in America, considering almost half of all calories Americans typically eat come from carbohydrates. What aren't taken into account when blindly blaming carbohydrates for obesity are portion sizes and the types of carbohydrates we typically eat. Many of the carbohydrates we consume have been processed to the point that they are stripped of their nutrients and fiber. Our bodies digest them quickly, leading to spikes in blood glucose and insulin in the blood stream, an occurrence now known to jeopardize your health.

Each time overly processed carbohydrates are eaten, blood-glucose levels rise sharply. To get rid of the glucose in your blood, the pancreas produces insulin. Insulin rids the blood of glucose, taking it to your muscles, where it can be used for energy. Consistent insulin release can have detrimental effects on the body, as insulin:

- Encourages the body to store calories as fat
- Promotes damage to the arteries
- May accelerate tumor growth
- Can encourage insulin resistance, a problem in which the body doesn't respond to insulin the way it should,

which is linked to obesity, high blood pressure, type II diabetes, and heart disease

Carbohydrates have typically been categorized as simple or complex, with complex carbohydrates being thought of as the healthier choice. These categories, however, tell us nothing about how the carbohydrates we eat affect our blood sugar and insulin levels. Research now suggests two better ways of distinguishing healthy from not-so-healthy carbohydrates:

- By whether they come from processed or whole grains
- By their effect on blood-glucose levels

The goal is to decrease the spikes in blood-glucose levels by eating more slowly digested carbohydrates. The measure of how different carbohydrates affect blood sugar is known as the Glycemic Index (GI). There are two commonly used indices. One uses glucose as a reference and randomly assigns it a GI of 100. The other uses white bread as a reference point, assigning it a GI of 100, which makes the GI of glucose 130. Using the index with the glucose GI of 100, foods with a GI of seventy or above are high-GI, those with a GI of fifty-six to sixty-nine are intermediate, and those with a GI of below fifty-six are low.

Food Type	GI
Breads	
Bagel	72
Croissant	67
"Grainy" breads	49
Pita bread	57
Rye bread	58
White bread	70

Food Type	GI
Legumes	
Baked beans	48
Broad beans	79
Butter beans	31
Chickpeas	28
Kidney beans	28
Lentils	29
Soy beans	18

(continued)

Food Type	GI		Food Type	GI
Dairy Foods			**Snack foods**	
Milk			Tortilla chips	63
Full fat	27		Peanuts	14
Skim	32		Popcorn	72
Chocolate flavored	42		Potato chips	57
Condensed	61		**Sugars**	
Ice cream			Honey	55
Regular	61		Fructose	19
Low fat	50		Glucose	100
Yogurt, low fat	33		Lactose	46
Fruit			Sucrose	68
Apple	38		**Sweets**	
Apricot	31		Chocolate	44
Banana	51		Doughnut, cake type	76
Cherries	22		Jelly beans	78
Grapefruit	25		**Vegetables**	
Grapes	46		Broccoli, raw	0
Kiwi	53		Carrots	47
Mango	51		Cauliflower	0
Orange	48		Celery	0
Papaya	59		Green peas	48
Peach	42		Lettuce	0
Pear	38		Potato	
Plum	39		—Baked	85
Raisins	64		—Boiled	88
Watermelon	72		—French fries	75
Grains/Pastas			Pumpkin	75
Buck wheat	54		Spinach	0
Bulgur	48		Sweet corn	60
Oatmeal, old-fashioned	42		Sweet potato	61
Rice			Rutabaga	72
Basamati	58		Yam	37
Brown	50			
Instant	87			
Pasta				
Spaghetti	38			
Vermicelli	35			

Excerpted from *The New Glucose Revolution*

The objective is not to restrict or eliminate carbohydrates but to be selective about which types you eat much of the time. Instead of eating white bread, cookies, and candy, make a conscious decision to eat fruits, vegetables, and whole-grain products with as much fiber as you can find. If you choose to eat a high-GI food, there are several things you can do to lower the GI of the overall meal, thus protecting yourself from the detrimental effects of excessive blood glucose and insulin:

- Add acid, such as vinegar, lemon juice, or an acidic fruit to your food
- Add healthy fats, such as olive oil or almond butter, to your food
- Balance a higher-GI carbohydrate, such as ready-to-eat cereal or white rice with a low-GI one, such as grapefruit or beans

Carbohydrates are the primary fuel for your body and brain and are necessary for healthy eating. To restrict them or eliminate them altogether is not only unrealistic, given our liking for carbohydrates, but it also ignores the research that points out the problem is not with all carbohydrates, but with the refined, processed ones we eat most frequently.

Fats

One message that Americans have heard loud and clear is "Fat is bad." Low-fat cookies and no-fat chips line the grocery-store shelves, and we spend billions of dollars on these products each year. Yet our weight has only increased.

> *In the United States, the gradual reduction in the fat content of the average diet, from 40 percent of calories to about 34 percent, has been accompanied by a gradual increase in the average weight and a dramatic increase in obesity.*
>
> —Walter C. Willett, M.D.

Three things the "fat is bad" message doesn't take into account are:

1. Some fat is essential to human function;
2. You will gain weight if you eat too many calories, regardless of how much or how little fat you consume; and
3. Not all fats are the same.

While fat in excess will cause weight gain, our bodies need some fat. Fat maintains healthy skin and hair; provides fuel for cells; helps create the material that protects our nerves; regulates blood pressure and cholesterol levels; helps us feel full and satisfied when we eat; and is a highly concentrated energy source, as it contains nine calories per gram, while carbohydrates and proteins contain four calories per gram.

Fats are typically categorized four ways: saturated, monounsaturated, polyunsaturated, and trans fat. See chart below for examples of each.

Dietary Fats

Monounsaturated	**Polyunsaturated**
Avocados Olives and olive oil Canola oil Peanuts, peanut butter, and peanut oil Cashews, almonds, and most other nuts and nut butters	Corn, soybean, safflower, and cottonseed oils Fatty fish Flaxseed, grapeseed, sunflower, and walnut oils
Saturated	**Trans**
Coconut, coconut oil and milk Palm and palm kernel oils Whole milk, butter, and cheese Red meat Chocolate	Margarine Partially-hydrogenated oils Vegetable shortening Most fast food Most commercial fried foods Most commercial baked goods

Unsaturated fats

These fats, including monounsaturated and polyunsaturated, remain liquid at room temperature and often originate from plant sources. Considered the healthy fats, eating unsaturated fats can:

- Improve cholesterol levels
- Help fight clogging of the arteries
- Decrease erratic heartbeats
- Prevent a rise in triglycerides, a fat that circulates in the bloodstream and has been linked with heart disease

Saturated fats

Saturated fats are abundant in animal protein, especially beef, dairy products, and palm and coconut oils. They are typically solid at room temperature and have been shown to increase levels of bad cholesterol (known as LDL or low-density lipoproteins), the prevalence of heart disease, and the risk of breast cancer.

Trans fats

Trans fats are vegetable oils that are processed to be thicker and more saturated, making them easier to ship and store. Trans fats are worse for you than saturated fats and currently exist in many of the foods we buy and eat every day. Check the labels on just about any package of chips, cookies, crackers, candy, or cereal and you'll find either partially hydrogenated oils or vegetable shortening, two ingredients loaded with trans fats. Trans fats are also abundant in fast food; fried food; commercial baked goods, such as bread, muffins, and donuts; and many frozen foods, such as fish sticks and pot pies.

The deceptive thing about trans fats is that they can currently be in many foods without being listed as fat on the nutrition label. For example, a product can show zero fat grams in its nutritional information, yet be made from hydrogenated oils, disguising the fact that it contains trans fat. This is why it's important to read the ingredients list of the products you eat. Fortunately, the government has told all food companies they must list trans-fat grams on nutrition labels by the year 2006, assuming the product contains more than .5 grams per serving.

Protein

Without enough protein, your nails and hair stop growing, wounds don't heal, and your muscle tissue breaks down. Most of the protein research has focused on the minimum amount needed for daily functioning, but not much exists on how much is too much or what is optimal for health. Despite what many diets and articles in muscle magazines suggest, the protein needs of most people are much lower than you think. Most people are nowhere near protein deficiency. Research suggests that adults need about one gram of protein per kilogram of weight daily. That's about eight grams of protein every day for every twenty pounds of weight. For a 180-pound woman that's seventy-two grams of protein daily.

Eating too much protein, on the other hand, has been linked to:

- Kidney disease
- Strain on the liver and kidneys
- Kidney stones
- Vitamin deficiency
- Decrease in muscle mass
- Bone loss
- Osteoporosis
- Gout
- Heart disease
- Cancer

Strategies for Success
Ditch Diets Completely

With dieting, decisions are made based solely on losing weight. Going forward, you want to base your decisions about food on health, respect for your body, and enjoyment. To be most effective with any plan you create, you must leave behind any remnants of dieting and the Diet Mindset, including any food rules you had previously adopted. This can take time and patience. Strive for an awareness of when the Diet Mindset appears. Success in living a healthy lifestyle takes flexibility and balance. Use of unrealistic food rules incorporates neither flexibility nor balance. One food rule I've heard frequently is to eat no later than three hours before your bedtime. While I'm not advocating eating a six-course meal before going to bed, if you're legitimately hungry, eat something. If you're eating enough throughout the day to support an active lifestyle and eating out of physical hunger, eating before bed will not become excessive.

Food rules are often put in place out of fear of doing something you don't want to do. Instead of taking responsibility for your behavior in a given situation, you put a rule in place to avoid the situation altogether. For example, there are a few common food rules based upon where you eat. The ones I've heard include: Not eating in your car, not eating while standing, and not eating while watching television. With rules, your life becomes inflexible. The goal is to make the best decisions for yourself, regardless of the situation.

WRITTEN EXERCISE

Food Rules

Instructions: One of the hardest things to let go of when moving to a healthy lifestyle is all of the food rules by which you live. It's important to let go of the rules, trusting yourself to make the decisions that are right for you in any situation. To do that, you must be aware of the rules you use. List all the food rules you have ever lived with below:

Read the Label

Reading food labels is critical to knowing what and how much you're eating. You'd be surprised to discover that what's packaged to look like a single serving is often much more than that. Be sure to check how many servings are included in the container. Also, notice the nutritional information is based on a single serving. So, if you choose to eat a whole package of food that has two servings, be sure to double all the information. What would be 250 calories in a single serving is now 500 calories if you eat the whole package.

Another important piece of the label is the ingredients list. Ingredients are listed in the order of amount in the product, with the first ingredient being the most prevalent. If whole wheat flour is listed as the first ingredient, the product consists mostly of whole wheat flour.

The ingredients list will give you information the nutrition label leaves out. For example, are the sugars in a product because it contains real fruit or because food manufacturers added high-fructose corn syrup to make the product sweeter? Or are there trans fats in something you're buying even though they aren't yet listed in the nutritional information?

Become a Conscious Eater

Many people, especially overeaters, have no idea how much they eat during the day. You have to know what the problems are before you can change them. It's hard to know where to start when you don't have the full picture. Tracking what, when, where, and how much you eat, as well as how you feel when you eat, gives you the full picture.

WRITTEN EXERCISE

On Your Way to Awareness

Instructions: Track what, how much, when, and where you eat, noting how you feel when you eat, for at least one full week. Don't allow the tracking to affect your eating behaviors. The goal is to get a realistic picture of how you currently eat. In a notebook or journal, start four columns with these headings:

What/how much—Write down everything you eat and drink every day. You want to track what and how much you eat of it, and you want to be as specific as possible. If you can measure it, measure it. If not, estimate the size.

When—Note the time next to every meal and snack you have. You want to know how long you go between meals, as well as when you eat what food.

Where—Write down where you're eating. Are you at home in front of the TV or at the dining-room table? Are you at work eating at your desk or eating out with friends?

How I feel—How do you feel when you're eating? You want to note your mood and how physically hungry you are. Are you guilty, anxious, or angry? Maybe you feel relaxed or even bored. And how hungry are you? Could you wait a while longer to eat, are you just starting to get hungry, or are you so hungry you could eat everything in sight?

Once the week is over, look at your journal for any patterns you think could be changed. Are you eating much more on the weekend than during the week? Do you eat breakfast? Are you eating a lot of junk food at work or late at night? Are you eating food off your children's plates? Was there a particular emotion that triggered a lot of eating for you?

In the left-hand column, make a list of what you'd like to change, using the middle column for any ideas you have to improve the pattern. Next, prioritize the things you want to focus on, labeling your most important item #1, your second most important item #2, etc. This will give you a realistic picture of where you are and will help determine where to start making improvements. An example has been included below.

Improvements	How to Improve	Priority
Example: I am ravenous at lunch because I don't eat anything until 11:30.	I will wake up a half an hour early to eat breakfast before work.	**#1**

Do What's Right for You

Determining what's right for you can be difficult after being told what to eat for so long. Even those who have never been on a diet struggle with guilt and remorse after eating a supposedly "bad" food. A woman will often say, "I've been bad today," as if she is now a bad person for having enjoyed the food she was eating. Yes, there are foods that are healthier than others, but losing weight is not about deprivation. It's about choices. It's about eating great-tasting, healthy foods. What you choose to eat and not eat is up to you. There is no authorized list of foods or someone telling you what you can and can't eat; the choice is yours.

For women who feel out of control when it comes to eating, this can be a frightening proposition. There's no longer someone telling you what to do or how to do it. You have to take full responsibility for your choices and believe that you can make the decisions that are right for you. Know that every healthy change you make is a step in the right direction. Be true to who you are and make decisions that are realistic for you.

As you begin to feel better about yourself and the choices you make, you'll find yourself making more choices out of respect for your body and your health.

Some Choices You Can Make

- Substitute not-so-healthy foods with healthier ones. Not only can you substitute various ingredients in the dishes you prepare, but you can substitute types of foods. For example, instead of getting your fats from beef, you may choose to get them from fish or beans instead.

- Cut down on portion sizes. If there are foods you can't imagine substituting, you can cut down on how much you eat of them in one sitting.

- Eat the foods you love less frequently. If you're used to eating ice cream every week, eat it twice a month instead. Eat the same amount you normally would and enjoy every bite.

- Eliminate a specific food or foods with a particular ingredient. For example, trans fats are the worst possible fats for your body. In an effort to eat more healthfully, you can choose similar products without hydrogenated oils. Instead of eating chocolate with caramel, which typically is made with trans fat, you could eat plain chocolate. You can also choose crackers, cereals, and chips that don't contain trans fat.

Develop a Game Plan

Many people go throughout the day giving little or no thought to what they eat and how it will affect their energy, productivity, and health.

If you want to eat most effectively, you must do some planning. How much planning is up to you. Some women like to plan each day's meals, leaving nothing to chance. However, some feel this approach to be too restrictive and not flexible enough for their lifestyles. Others, knowing they eat healthfully at home, plan ahead only for those times they won't be home to eat. Whatever your approach, it must be based on your lifestyle for it to be effective. Do you travel a lot for work? Do you not like to cook? Do you typically cook meals for your whole family? Take these things into account when thinking about what you'll eat for the week.

> *A Restaurant and Institutions survey showed that 70 percent of Americans don't even think about what to eat for dinner until after 4:00 P.M.*

Healthful Hints

- Take emotional triggers into account when developing a game plan. When are you most likely to eat for reasons other than physical hunger?
- Create a grocery list and buy only those items.
- Go to the grocery store on a full stomach. You're more likely to buy not-so-healthy food when you're hungry.
- Stick to the aisles with the healthiest food. Why tempt yourself by walking down the junk-food aisles?
- Shop at a health food store periodically. They often have a greater variety of organic products, nuts, and seeds.
- Check and compare food labels.
- Be willing to try new things.
- Prepare healthy food ahead of time, so it's ready and waiting when you're hungry.
- Have healthy snacks for yourself and your family at all times. You'll be less likely to grab a quick, unhealthy bite to eat on the commute home from work, on the way to the gym, or while running errands with the kids.

WRITTEN EXERCISE

Challenges to Eating Healthfully

Instructions: Make a list of all the things you consider challenges to eating healthfully. Next to each item, write your action plan to deal with the challenge.

Challenge	Action Plan
Example: I am responsible for buying groceries and cooking for everyone in my family.	I will buy healthy food and cook healthy meals for everyone, so that we all can eat more healthfully. I will discuss this with them and get their ideas and suggestions when I tell them about my plan.

Go at Your Own Pace

A common mistake women make when changing their eating habits is believing they must change their behaviors all at once. This is not the case. The best approach is to make gradual changes to your eating behaviors, adding a new change when ready. This increases the likelihood that the new behaviors will be permanent. Eating healthfully does not require an all-or-nothing approach. Every positive change brings you closer to your overall objective of eating healthfully for a lifetime.

Recognize Portion Distortion

Did you know that portions in the U.S. have grown two to five times larger than they were thirty years ago? The amount of food we're served in restaurants and find in grocery stores has caused us to lose perspective about what an appropriate portion size is. Many restaurants serve meals that contain a full day's worth of calories. Research shows we eat significantly more as our serving sizes increase.

So, What Is a Portion?

A great way to approximate a portion is to use the size of your palm for fish, poultry, and meats; use your clenched fist for vegetables and whole grains; and think of a tennis ball to determine the appropriate portions for yogurt, cottage cheese, and whole pieces of fruit.

> *In a recent American Institute for Cancer Research (AICR) survey, 70 percent of the respondents said they ate whatever amount they were served in a restaurant most of the time.*

Serving Size Success Strategies

In a restaurant:

- Get the smallest size available; do not supersize.
- Share one meal or dessert with friends.
- Determine a portion and get the rest to take home.

In the grocery store and at home:

- Read labels to determine how many servings are in a package.
- Buy products in single-serving sizes, when available.
- When buying something with multiple servings, break it down into single-serving-size containers.

Eat Consistently Throughout the Day

Many people eat haphazardly, at best. They skip breakfast, eat a huge lunch after going all morning without food, snack whenever the feeling strikes, and come home to eat a big dinner and late-night snack.

Food is the fuel that keeps your body going. If you're tired during the day, can't concentrate, or suffer from frequent headaches, lack of food and water may be the issue. Eating five to six small meals throughout the day, starting with breakfast, keeps energy levels consistent and helps you get the nutrients your body needs. It also curbs overeating, as you're never starving between meals. Current research also suggests eating more frequently helps keep blood-sugar levels consistent.

Research done for The Journal of the American Dietetic Association found that more than half of the overweight women in the study conducted ate 70 percent of their daily calories after 7:00 P.M.

Eating many small meals a day can be hard to accomplish, especially if you aren't even used to eating three consistent meals a day. Your first step is to eat regularly throughout the day, regardless of how many meals you have. For some, this may mean scheduling food breaks every three to four hours to ensure you eat. For others, it means learning to pay attention to the hunger signals your body gives you before you're so hungry you could eat everything in sight. If you feel eating five or six small meals is unrealistic for you, aim for three or four.

A Calorie Is Not Just a Calorie

Many weight-loss experts would have you believe that weight loss is as easy as eating fewer calories than what you burn. While this is important, what you eat is equally as important for long-term results. Exercise is an integral part in maintaining a healthy body weight. To fuel your body for exercise you must eat more healthy food and less not-so-healthy food. Potato chips and ice cream will barely get you through a day of sitting at a desk, let alone exercising enough to change the way you look and feel. And, remember, you can look thin and still be at risk of serious illness due to lack of healthy eating. Eating well can influence your health, change the way you feel about yourself and your body, and bring pleasure to your life.

What's Best?
Do I Need to Count Calories?

Numerous studies show overweight people consistently underestimate the number of calories they eat by one-half. That's a lot of calories that are unaccounted for. The problems usually lie in eating portions that are too big and eating foods that are high in calories. Eating proper portion sizes and substituting healthier foods for not-so-healthy ones will start you in the right direction. As you progress, you will learn how much food is right for you.

For those of you who consistently eat too many calories, despite making healthy changes, it may be useful to get a realistic calorie count for your height, weight, and activity level, and count calories for a week or two to determine how much you're truly eating. Just type "How many calories do I need?" on any search engine, and it will take you to numerous calorie counters. Others of you, especially those looking for more direction, may like the structure that counting calories provides. Remember that while counting calories can be an educational tool, it can also become one that's used to hold you to a rigid standard. Flexibility and balance must be part of any plan for it to last a lifetime.

What About Supplements?

In our pill-oriented, quick-fix society, there is a pill for just about every ailment. Have a headache? Take a pill. Have heartburn? Take a pill. Have high cholesterol? Take a pill. What about addressing the causes of your heartburn or headaches, as opposed to masking them with medications?

The same goes for weight-loss supplements. Instead of addressing the causes for weight gain, many women take pills as a quick fix, hoping their fat will just melt away. Some women take supplements to speed the weight-loss process or because they don't believe they can lose weight on their own. Very few supplements, if any, do all they say they will. Some do nothing at all and some are detrimental to your health, even deadly (e.g., ephedra).

It is important that you research any supplement before taking it, so you are well aware of what you are putting into your body.

Healthy Steps

1. Eat lots of fruits and vegetables. Get in as many as you can, aiming for a minimum of five servings daily. Aim for variety in type and color, with darker being more nutri-

tious. Add fruits and vegetables to your main dishes, use them as colorful side dishes or as a dessert, and eat them as snacks. Eating fruits and vegetables can:

- Lower the likelihood of heart disease, heart attack, and stroke·
- Decrease blood pressure
- Guard against cancer
- Protect against two common eye diseases—cataracts and macular degeneration
- Add variety and flavor to food

2. Increase your intake of unrefined, high-fiber, low-GI carbohydrates. Most Americans get less than one serving of whole-grain foods a day. Whole-grain products are rich in vitamins, minerals, carbohydrates, and fiber. Instead we eat processed, easily digested foods, which are stripped of their fiber and nutrients and injected with sugar, fat, salt, and preservatives. Start eating whole-grain breads, cereals, and pastas, instead of white bread, pasta, and rice. Use whole wheat flour when baking and add seeds to pancakes, oatmeal, and homemade muffins and breads.

> *One-fourth of all vegetables eaten in the United States are French fries.*
> —Source: *Food Fight*

3. Decrease your overall fat consumption, while substituting saturated and trans fats with unsaturated ones. Despite all the low-fat and no-fat products lining grocery-store shelves, two-thirds of American women get more than 30 percent of their daily calories from fat. With fat containing nine calories per gram, it doesn't take much to overeat.

If you are one of these women, your first step is to determine where you can decrease and eliminate fat from your eating plan. Common sources include the sauces and

condiments we add to our foods such as butter, marga-
rine, cheese, and salad dressing. Other sources include
full-fat dairy products and meat. Try low-fat or no-fat milk,
cheese, and yogurt. You can also try veggie cheese or soy
milk. Substitute beans, nuts, tofu, and fish for beef or
chicken. If you enjoy eating meat, opt for lean chicken
and turkey or wild game, such as buffalo or venison. Decrease your intake of fast food and popular snack foods,
such as potato chips, ice cream, and chocolate.

4. Pay attention to how much sugar you eat. The average
American woman consumes 158 pounds of sugar each
year. That's forty-three teaspoons daily. Read labels to
determine where your sugar is coming from. Beyond the
sweet treats we typically associate with sugar, common
sources include cereal, yogurt, and juice. There are four
grams of sugar in a teaspoon, so a yogurt containing
twenty-six grams of sugar equals six and one-half teaspoons. Add up your sugar intake; you may be surprised.

5. Be sure you're getting enough water. Water is the most
abundant nutrient in your body, making up 70 to 75 percent of your total body weight. It aids in digestion, keeps
joints lubricated, allows your blood to deliver oxygen to
your brain and muscles, regulates your body temperature,
and is vital to your survival. The general rule of thumb is
to drink eight glasses of water daily, but this number goes
up to nine to thirteen if you exercise regularly.

6. Spice it up and be willing to try new things. Use spicy
mustards, low-salt salsas, herbs, and spices to keep your
food interesting. They add flavor to your food without
the salt, sugar, fat, and additives found in commercial and
homemade sauces and dressings. You may just discover
you like tuna fish without mayonnaise or broccoli that's
not drowning in cheese sauce.

7. If you drink alcohol, drink it in moderation. Alcohol contains seven calories per gram, almost as much as fat, yet provides no nutrients, doesn't fill you up, and slows your metabolism. Further, most of what people eat while drinking alcohol is junk food filled with fat, sugar, and salt. And alcohol does nothing to encourage a challenging workout.

Wrap-Up

There is no one right way to eat. I have done my best to share the latest research and provide healthful options, while leaving the choices up to you. You must trust yourself to make the food decisions that are realistic and healthy for you.

> *Eating well simply means using a basic understanding of human nutrition to maximize as much as you can both the nourishing and pleasure-giving qualities of food.*
>
> —Andrew Weil, M.D.

CHAPTER 3

I Will Do It!

CREATING YOUR OWN CUSTOMIZED PLAN

The Importance of Having a Plan

Most of us spend more time planning our vacations than planning what we consider most important in our lives—our families, our careers, our health. Accomplishing lifelong health and quality of life requires focus on what you want to achieve and a commitment to doing what it takes to achieve it. A plan will facilitate that focus and help drive your decisions in life. When you know what you want and have a plan to get there, it's easier to do what's necessary to achieve your goals.

We often live our lives with no thought as to where our actions will take us. We base our decisions on our mood at that moment or the particular situation, as opposed to the results we ultimately want to achieve. It's not that we want the results we're getting; it's

> *Anything less than a conscious commitment to the important is an unconscious decision to the unimportant.*
> —Stephen R. Covey

that we didn't plan for the results we wanted in the first place.

Life will continue whether or not you have a plan. By creating and following a plan, you make a conscious decision to live the life you want to live.

Start With Your Key Objectives

What are the first things that come to your mind when asked what you want to accomplish from reading this book? These are likely your key objectives. When thinking of your objectives, you want to think of your longer-term, less-specific, all-encompassing goals. For example, you may want to reach a healthy body weight. This is a key objective.

Setting objectives gives you a basic understanding of what you want to accomplish without getting into the details. It's the starting point for creating and achieving effective weekly goals.

Strategies for Successful Objective Setting
Set Objectives While Asking How and Why

Asking why you want to accomplish something and how you want to accomplish it helps determine whether you're doing the right things for the right reasons and in the right ways for you. It ensures that you'll set goals that will achieve quality-of-life results.

Set At Least One Objective for Each Dimension of Health

To create the most beneficial and effective plan for you, you must address each dimension of health. Creating an objective for each dimension ensures each is included in your plan.

WRITTEN EXERCISE

Setting Your Objectives

Instructions: Set an objective (a "What") for each dimension below (P-Physical, M-Mental, Sp-Spiritual, S-Social), while asking yourself why you want to do it and how to accomplish it. Review page 36 for a list of possible objectives for each dimension. An example is included below.

Example:

Dimension:	**Social**
What:	Create a comprehensive support network.
Why:	I'm more likely to achieve my goals when surrounded by people who support my efforts.
	It's an opportunity to better my relationships by sharing goals and involving family and friends whenever possible.
How:	Have meetings with family and friends to share my goals and ask for their help.

P

What:

Why:

How:

M

What:

Why:

How:

Sp
What:

Why:

How:

───

S
What:

Why:

How:

Rethink and Review Objectives Regularly

As you accomplish your objectives, set new ones. As you become better at objective setting, your objectives may change. It's OK to desert a good objective for a better one.

As time passes, it's easy to lose sight of why you're doing what you're doing. A weekly review of your objectives, why you want to the achieve them, and how you plan to achieve them will keep you on track.

> *So often, the enemy of the best is the good.*
> —Stephen R. Covey

Start a Possibilities List

A possibilities list is just that—possibilities. It is a list of possible objectives without the commitment of having to achieve them. If you've always thought it would be great to run a marathon, join a volleyball league, or take an active vacation but you aren't ready to commit to the ideas, add them to your possibilities list. This way, you can keep track of any objective ideas you have without putting your integrity on the line.

When reviewing your objectives, keep your list of possibilities readily accessible. You can add them to your plan as objectives, keep them on your list for future consideration, or remove them from the list as you see fit.

Weekly Goals

Why Weekly?

Goal setting to many means creating a daily "to-do" list. Having only daily goals doesn't allow you to see the big picture. It limits your focus to what's urgent, as opposed to what's most important in achieving your objectives. It keeps you so much in the present and focused on that day that it's hard to plan for the future.

Organizing your entire week provides context for your daily achievements and allows flexibility and balance in your schedule. Instead of getting lost in the efficiency and urgency of the day, your daily activities take on more meaning when determined with your weekly goals and key objectives in mind. You are spending time on what really matters, as opposed to day-to-day busy work.

Breaking Down the "How"

You now have at least one objective for each dimension of health and know how you're going to achieve that objective. The next step is to break down your "hows" to create weekly goals. Using the example from the previous exercise, one of your "hows" is to set up a meeting with your family to discuss your goals and ask for their help. To break it down further, you want to think about and write down all the steps necessary for an effective family meeting. I have provided possible steps below:

1. Collect information on family members' free time, so I can schedule a meeting that everyone can attend.
2. Schedule a meeting and make sure everyone knows it's important to be there.
3. Think about what I'll say to best communicate my plan's importance.
4. Think about possible questions from my family and be prepared to respond.
5. Prepare for any resistance to my plan.

Each step then becomes a weekly goal. Remember to be realistic with your time and focus only on what you can accomplish in a given week.

Strategies for Successful Goal Setting
Allow Your Values to Drive Your Goals
The best goals reflect your deep needs and desires for quality of life. They don't reflect a social image or what others want for you. Make sure you create goals based upon what is most important to you and reflective of your true identity.

Strive for Overall Balance
While setting at least one weekly goal from each dimension will help with balance and effective planning, it is not necessary to set a goal in each dimension every week. There may be times that warrant purposeful, short-term imbalance. The aim is to nurture each dimension in the long term.

Keep Goals Realistic, Yet Challenging
This can be difficult to achieve initially. If you have never created such a plan and don't know what you're capable of, it's easy to set goals that don't challenge your body. On the

other hand, in your enthusiasm to get started, it's also easy to find yourself overwhelmed with too many demanding goals. It's particularly important in the initial weeks that you review your goals and strike a balance that is both realistic and challenging. I will discuss evaluating your plan later in this section of the book.

Set Behavior-Focused Goals

How many times have you set a goal such as, "I will lose twenty pounds by my high school reunion" or "I want to be a size six by the end of the year"? These goals are weight-focused, they are often unrealistic, and they say nothing about how you plan to achieve the weight loss.

While there's nothing wrong with setting a realistic goal weight, setting weight-related goals focuses on a symptom of the problem (the weight), as opposed to the cause of the problem (too little exercise and too much food). Further, weight-related goals set you up for failure. While you can choose how you treat your body, exactly how or how fast your body responds to that treatment varies from woman to woman. Trying to achieve such goals can be unrealistic and self-defeating. Instead, set behavior-focused goals, such as biking for twenty minutes three days a week or eating an additional serving of vegetables every day. These goals focus on the cause of the problem, address changing your behavior, are within your control, and are easily measurable, since you either do them or you don't.

Take Back Your Time

Once you have identified your goals, it's critical to schedule time for them. This, too, may take practice, depending upon how you currently spend your time. Many women allow the urgency or flow of the day to take over, often accomplishing nothing of true importance day after day. They do only those things that are most convenient, easiest, or that they're receiving pressure from someone else to do. Sound familiar?

If you have a current list of "to-dos," look at it now. When I've had women do this, their common response is "But I have to do the laundry" or "I have to go to work." The truth is, you don't *have to* do anything on your list; you make a choice to do what you do during the day. The question is, are your choices in alignment with what is most important to you? If not, it's time to rethink how you spend your time. You want to schedule your priorities, spending the majority of each day on what you value most. What you don't want to do is be a slave to your schedule, scheduling every second of your day. This doesn't allow for flexibility to respond to those things that are truly urgent or simply more important than what you have planned. You want to use your schedule to achieve your goals, while remaining available for unplanned opportunities.

> *If something is on their To Do list, it has the same importance as anything else on the list, but petty chores do not deserve the same attention as a major dream. It's up to each of us to identify our true priorities and then align ourselves with the highest and best on the list.*
>
> —David Viscott, Ph.D.

WRITTEN EXERCISE

Got Time?

Instructions: Write out your typical schedule below, noting as many details as possible. You may want to do separate schedules for week days and weekend days.

Once your schedule is complete, review it while highlighting or circling the free time you have. This will allow you to see the time you do have available. It may also indicate a need to reprioritize your time to make a commitment to your health.

Combine Goals, When It Makes Sense

The number one reason given for not exercising is lack of time. Why not combine your exercise and nutrition goals with another goal? This way, you save time and get both goals accomplished. You may even find that combining goals leads to a better experience or more opportunities than if each goal had been achieved separately. For example, you want to spend more time with your daughter. You also want to exercise, but you only have an hour in your day. Why not go on a walk with your daughter? This way, you work on your relationship, do something good for your body, and instill healthy habits in your daughter by being an excellent role model.

WRITTEN EXERCISE

Creative Combining

Instructions: To combine exercise and nutrition with what is most important to you, you must determine what is most important. This is the time to get creative and focus on ways you can "fit" fitness and nutrition into your life. Think about your other key goals, as well as what you do day to day. Take time to list your most important goals in the left-hand column below. In the right-hand column, list creative ways to combine your goals with your active lifestyle. Several examples have been included below.

Goals	How to Combine
Examples:	
1. Spend more time with my family.	Hike with my husband and children two times a week. Cook Sunday-morning breakfast as a family. Walk my daughter to school three times a week.
2. Improve business knowledge.	Listen to books on tape while working out or cooking.

Make Goal Setting a Lifelong Habit

Goal-setting, as with living a fit lifestyle, is a lifelong process. In order to keep achieving, you must keep setting goals. Without goals, it's easy to get caught up in doing the unimportant and lose sight of what matters most to you. This happens frequently once women have lost weight. The weight is gone and you have no plan to keep it off, so it creeps back on.

> *When you don't know where you're going, you're likely to get there.*
>
> —Unknown

WRITTEN EXERCISE

Setting Your Goals

Instructions: Using your "hows" as a guide, list any goals you think of below. List as many as you can, without censoring them.

Once your list is complete, be sure to:

- Check to see your goals meet the "Strategies for Successful Goal Setting" criteria on page 100.
- Eliminate or reword those that don't meet the criteria.
- Prioritize them according to what is most important to you.
- Add them to your plan.

Keep Promises to Yourself

When you determine a goal and write it down, it becomes a promise. Your intent is to accomplish that goal. With each promise you keep, you build self-esteem, confidence, and a belief that you can follow through despite the obstacles. With each promise kept, more becomes possible.

How many times have you set goals either to start and give up or to never start at all? How did you feel about yourself afterward? My guess is, not very good. Make these goals the promises you keep to yourself. Take responsibility for your life and health, and then follow through. You know you'll feel better about yourself when you do.

Working Your Plan

Now that you've determined your objectives and weekly goals, it's time to take action.

Strategies for Success

Get Moving

Since you never know what you'll encounter until you get started...get started. This process is learn-as-you-go. You don't have to plan it all to get started, nor will it ever be the perfect time. Just start.

> *If we wait for the moment when everything, absolutely everything is ready, we shall never begin.*
> —Ivan Turgenev

Give It Time to Work

In the world of diets, you're used to seeing changes in your body quickly. But, remember, the weight always comes back. Be sure to give yourself the time to do things the right way. Quick weight-loss results, at the expense of your long-term health or permanent weight loss, are not what you want when changing your lifestyle to a healthy one. Instead, focus on the changes that *are* occurring, such as how much better you feel physically, the fact that you have more energy, or that you feel great about doing something good for yourself. Focus on changing your identity, not chasing an image.

Evaluate Your Results

You've created your plan and have been following it for a couple months now. Have you achieved what you want? What obstacles did you encounter? Were all of your goals both realistic and challenging? Do you know the answers to these questions?

Even when women manage to set health goals, they rarely look back to evaluate the results. If they get the results they want—great. If not, they quit trying without determining what went wrong. Weekly evaluation is critical to learning what did and didn't work and to holding yourself accountable to creating your best plan possible.

How to Evaluate Weekly

Evaluation can be done wherever you track your goals and should be completed before setting goals for the following week. When evaluating your previous week, you want to review your goals while asking several questions. You can determine your own questions or choose from the list below. Use your evaluation to plan the following week.

- What goals did I accomplish?
- What helped me accomplish them?
- What obstacles did I face?
- How can I overcome such obstacles in the future?
- Did I accomplish the right things for the right reasons in the right ways?
- Did my goals reflect my objectives?
- Is my plan taking me where I want to go?
- What goals didn't I accomplish?
- What kept me from achieving my goals?
- Should I add my unmet goals to my plan for next week?

- Was I able to combine goals?
- Did combining goals create a better experience than if they had been achieved separately? Why or why not?
- How do I feel about last week?
- What would make me feel better about the upcoming week?
- What can I learn from last week?

Seeing the Big Picture

As time progresses, you will want to evaluate your plan on a monthly, quarterly, or yearly basis asking yourself these questions:

- Am I getting the results I want?
- Are my goals both realistic and challenging?
- What patterns am I seeing that I want to continue?
- What patterns do I want to stop?
- Are there any obstacles that keep appearing?
- What else can I change?

> *Obstacles are those frightful things you see when you take your eyes off your goal.*
>
> —Henry Ford

WRITTEN EXERCISE

Overcoming Your Obstacles

Instructions: In the left-hand column, list the obstacles that you still face. In the right-hand column, list any ideas you have to overcome each obstacle An example is below.

Obstacles	Ideas to Overcome Obstacle
Example: Cold weather	Buy warmer exercise clothing. Learn to snowshoe or cross-country ski. Buy new CDs to keep me motivated when working out indoors.

Make Your Plan Distinctly Yours

The best plan is the one you'll commit to and follow. Don't rely solely on others to tell you what to eat, when to exercise, or what exercise equipment to use. You are an individual with distinct likes and dislikes, obstacles, motivators, and objectives. Educate yourself, determine what works best for you, and trust yourself to make the right decisions.

CHAPTER 4

I Am Doing It!
STAYING MOTIVATED WHEN ALL YOU WANT TO DO IS QUIT

The First Six Weeks

When starting to exercise and eat healthfully, staying motivated for the first six weeks is critical to long-term success.

Being prepared for the following obstacles will help.

Uncomfortable, Self-conscious, and Embarrassed

Research shows that 80 percent of people stop what they're doing within six weeks.

Don't be surprised if you feel all three, particularly if you haven't exercised in some time or aren't feeling great about your body. Keep this in mind when getting started, and recognize how you respond to these feelings. Whatever you do, don't give up.

There are too many options available to allow these feelings to hamper your efforts. If you feel uncomfortable being seen by others, consider working out at home to videotapes, hiring a personal trainer for one-on-one sessions, or visiting the gym at off-peak times. Try a women-only gym if you feel more comfortable. If you go to a gym, focus only on yourself. Focus on how your body feels when it's moving, watch the TV, or jam to your music. Go with a friend who will keep you focused on what's important—you and your health. Do whatever it takes to get you past these initial feelings of awkwardness. They will pass.

> *That which we persist in doing becomes easier to do.*
>
> —Ralph Waldo Emerson

Fluctuations in Weight

You will have fluctuations in your weight due to changes in water weight. And the heavier you are, the more your weight can change from day to day. Some of these fluctuations can be quite large, causing you to question if what you're doing is working. For those of you who allow your weight to define success or failure, I strongly suggest hiding the scale at this point; forget it exists. Instead, focus on how good it feels to work out and take care of yourself. Do the right things out of respect for your body and have faith the fat will come off. Remind yourself that the ultimate goal is not to lose weight but to live a healthy lifestyle, and the rest will take care of itself.

> *Have trust in yourself and the process—the weight will come off.*

I'm Not Seeing the Results I Want

The "first on, last off" rule describes how body fat responds to exercise. The places you first started gaining fat (usually hips, thighs, and butt), the places you most want to lose the fat quickly, are the places that usually lose fat last. Expect this and expect that it will be frustrating, but don't allow the frustration to stop your journey. It isn't that your plan isn't working; it's just how body fat works. Stay focused on the positive effects of exercise and have faith the fat will come off.

Not all benefits of exercise are visible in the mirror. How do you feel? Do you have more energy? Are you sleeping better? Don't negate all the benefits you're experiencing because you don't see any changes in how your body looks. Take a look at the big picture. After just one cardiovascular workout, you will experience several psychological benefits: better mood, increased relaxation, decreased anxiety, and an increase in self-esteem and confidence. Every workout benefits your body and your long-term health. Don't give up.

Muscle Soreness

When a muscle experiences more intense exercise than usual or an unfamiliar exercise, it often ends up sore. However, the soreness doesn't occur right away, which can be deceiving. You feel great during your workout, and then twenty-four to forty-eight hours later, you're in pain and feeling as though you never want to work out again. When starting something new, be sure to take it slowly. The time to push yourself is when you have more experience. As your body becomes more fit, take solace in the fact that soreness will occur less frequently.

If you do end up sore, this is not the time to stop exercising out of fear you'll end up more sore or hurt. The best way to alleviate the pain is to do a less-intense version of the same exercise that caused the soreness initially.

I'm Sick!

You were all excited about exercising and now you're sick. When you first become active, your body is not used to the new challenge and may become ill. This is not the time to give up completely. Focus on the non-physical parts of your plan. Have you had your family meeting yet? Are there changes in your environment you could be making? Maybe you could read a book on nutrition or stock your shelves with healthy food.

If you're thinking about exercising anyway, check with your doctor.

A Perfect Time to Journal

Journaling is a great way to work through obstacles, analyze your choices, highlight your healthy decisions, and write about how strong you feel after lifting weights. When changing your lifestyle to a healthy one, each day presents unexpected challenges, opportunities for learning, and excuses for not following through on your plan. There will be days you don't want to work out or times when all you want to eat is junk food. Journaling is the perfect way to capture these experiences and learn from them.

- What situations did you encounter today?
- What choices did you make? Were they healthy or not-so-healthy? Did your goals drive the decisions you made?
- How do you feel about the choices you made?
- How are you feeling as you're journaling? Are you exhausted and frustrated, feeling uncertain about your plan? Or, despite the challenges, do you feel good about the choices you made and look forward to tomorrow?

Do What It Takes

Use these first six weeks to try new things, learn what you like and don't like, and do whatever it takes to get to the seventh week. There are so many excuses women use to allow themselves to give up. Recognize them for what they are—excuses—and continue with your plan.

WRITTEN EXERCISE

So Many Excuses

Instructions: As you progress through this period, write down in the left-hand column the excuses you use for not making healthy choices. In the right-hand column, challenge each one. Examples are included below.

Excuses	Challenge
Example: 1. I was so hungry, I had to stop at McDonald's on the way home.	I could have had healthy food in my car with me.
2. I was just too tired to work out.	Exercise leaves me feeling invigorated; I could have started, and stopped if I felt too tired to continue.

WRITTEN EXERCISE

Motivators

Instructions: For the next six weeks, write down everything that kept you motivated to follow through on your plan. Note which motivators you used most frequently and which are most effective. Use this list beyond the six-week period to keep you going. Examples are included below.

Examples:

1. Instead of getting on the treadmill again today, I tried the elliptical machine at the gym.

2. I visualized what I would look and feel like once I reach a healthy weight.

Possible Motivators

Here's a list of several motivators that may apply to you. Feel free to try any of them.

1. Celebrate your successes when you meet goals.
2. Post your goals where you can see them every day.
3. Build a comprehensive support system that includes friends, family, pets, and professionals.
4. Play your favorite music.
5. Try something new.
6. Challenge yourself.
7. Educate yourself about exercise and healthy eating.
8. Buy new workout clothes.
9. Join a gym.
10. Join an aerobics class.
11. Invest in a personal trainer or nutritionist.
12. Head outdoors.
13. Work out for a cause (e.g., breast cancer, diabetes, AIDS).
14. Tie exercise to other things you enjoy (e.g., if you like to travel, go on an active vacation).
15. Focus on how good you feel after your workout. Write those feelings down, and hang them up for motivation.
16. Keep a training log to note your progress.
17. Compete with yourself.
18. Read motivational books or magazines.
19. Choose activities with a purpose (e.g., walk to the grocery store to pick up food or bike to work).
20. Change other aspects of your life (e.g., hairstyle, wardrobe).
21. Use the ten-minute rule (i.e., when all you feel like doing is plopping down on the couch to watch TV, force yourself to exercise for ten minutes. If after ten minutes, you still don't want to work out, stop.)

There are so many things you can do to keep yourself motivated. Tap into the ones that work best for you. If you think of others not listed above, please share them with me at www.trustyourselftotransform.com.

After the First Six Weeks

Celebrate

Congratulations! You've done something 80 percent of people don't. You've made it to the six-week mark. Take time to celebrate what you've accomplished.

Look Back and Learn

Now that the six weeks are over, it's time to learn from your experience. In evaluating the last six weeks, you want to ask yourself some questions:

- What kept you motivated throughout this process?
- What are the obstacles you faced?
- What can you do to overcome them going forward?
- Do you foresee any future obstacles?
- What worked and what didn't?
- What would you like to continue, stop, or start doing in this process?
- Overall, what did you learn from the last six weeks that you can apply in the future?

Making Changes

Instructions: Now that you've gotten to the six-week mark, there may be things you want to change in your life to better support your healthy lifestyle. Do you eat out weekly with friends or your husband? Or, maybe, you watch several hours of television a day. Make a list in the left-hand column of everything you need to change and write in the right-hand column alternatives to that behavior. These are changes you want to include in your plan.

Change	Alternative
Example: I currently watch three or four hours of TV a day.	I will watch only two hours of TV a day, using my free time to exercise and spend time with my family.

Body Boredom

The biggest obstacle to overcome is sticking with your plan once you've stopped seeing the results you desire. This is often when people get frustrated and give up. Don't you dare give up. Assuming you're sticking to your plan, this means your body has adapted to your current workout, and you are making progress. This is a good thing.

> *Effort only fully releases its reward after a person refuses to quit.*
>
> —Napoleon Hill

The secret to minimizing plateaus is to consistently work variety into your plan. In the beginning, you want to make sure you have fully mastered any exercise before you add another one. This will ensure proper technique and minimize injury. Depending upon your experience and your body's need for variety, you will want to change your routine every three to six weeks.

When you hit a plateau, use the time to experiment with new things and learn about your body. When your weight becomes stable, you know how much exercise and food you need to maintain your current weight. This knowledge can be helpful when you no longer want to lose weight.

Getting Past Body Boredom

Take a closer look at what you're doing for any signs of self-sabotage. Assuming you're sticking to your plan, it's time for a change. Here are some ways to mix it up:

With aerobics, you can vary:
- The length of your workout
- The frequency you workout
- The intensity of your work out
- The type of exercise you do

With strength training, you can vary:

- The amount of weight you use
- The order of exercises within your routine, as long as you continue to work larger muscles first
- How often you train
- The number of repetitions for each exercise
- The number of sets for each exercise
- The type of exercise for each body part
- The equipment you use

Creating a Lifelong Habit

As you continue to experiment with exercise and nutrition, focus on what you enjoy most and update your goals and objectives to reflect what you learn. If something isn't working, change it. As you try new things, you'll want to determine what you are and aren't willing to do to maintain your healthy lifestyle.

Realize the decisions you make when motivated by weight loss can be quite different from those motivated by long-term health. It's easier to practice extreme behaviors in the interest of losing weight. You get excited by the results you're seeing, so you exercise a little more and eat a little less than you would on a long-term basis. Yes, some behaviors you choose when losing weight are going to be different from those you select once you've lost the weight. However, you want to make decisions based upon living healthfully and your long-term goals. Creating a lifelong habit requires flexibility, balance, and an ability to maintain your lifestyle.

Tiana's Story

My weight became an issue at age twelve when I weighed 140 pounds. I went on antidepressants at age fifteen to help with obsessive-compulsive disorder, and gained more weight. By the year 2000, I was at 260 pounds. At age twenty-three, I weighed 296 pounds, the most I had ever weighed.

I've tried the fast-fix diet, starving-yourself thing. It worked for a few months, and then I started eating again. I wanted to get gastric bypass surgery. My family and I fought and fought over it. A friend of mine had gotten it and started losing weight. I was so jealous.

My attitude changed when I joined the gym and saw a girl I had gone to high school with. She was always overweight and made fun of. She had lost over 100 pounds on her own. In her own way, she was saying, *You can do it, too.*

I've lost 100 pounds so far and have forty more pounds to lose. I've done it on my own—no diets, no pills, no surgery—just working out and watching what I eat. It has become a habit. The main key in doing this is learning how food and exercise go hand in hand. It's also accepting you're not going to lose 100 pounds in five months. It took me about a year to lose the first seventy pounds. I took my time starting to work out and cutting back on my food a slight amount. By the time I was 230 pounds, I was so used to everything, I was ready to go for it all.

When people say it's a life change, they are understating what it really is. I feel it's a *person* change. You are changing everything about yourself—the way you look at the world and at yourself.

CHAPTER 5

I Did It!

NOW WHAT?

.

But Wait...There's More

I struggled in deciding what to call this chapter. "I Did It!" communicates a finality to the process, a message I wasn't sure I wanted to give. But it also communicates a well-deserved acknowledgment of all you have achieved thus far. This, I definitely wanted to communicate.

You have accomplished what you set out to do. It's time to recognize all you have achieved and realize there is still much more you can achieve. What once seemed impossible is now possible. Each new achievement creates new opportunity. Each step taken makes another step a reality.

WRITTEN EXERCISE

Why Stay Healthy?

Instructions: List all the reasons it's important for you to stay fit and healthy below. Pull out this list when your motivation is low. Or hang it up where you'll see it every day to remind you of the importance of health in your life.

So Much More Than Weight Loss

You probably started reading this book with the goal of losing weight. My hope is that you now realize this process is about so much more than that. It's about feeling good about the decisions you make, about caring enough about yourself and your health to make the decisions that are right for you, about keeping promises to yourself and others, and about living a lifestyle that allows you to be your best you.

As you progress, living healthfully becomes less about what it takes to lose weight and more about living your best life possible. It comes to encompass all areas of your life—your family, your career, and your relationships with others and yourself. You want more for yourself, and you believe that more is possible.

A key piece to remember is that living healthfully can mean different things to different women. In fact, the definition of living healthfully will change for you over time, so that what you were doing a week, a month, or a year ago may have changed or stopped altogether. Living healthfully is a process, a lifelong process you can adjust to your needs, goals, and situation.

What Does Living Healthfully Mean to You Now?

Instructions: Take time to note what you consider to be part of a healthy lifestyle. Next to each item, place a ✔ if the item is something you already do, or a **0** if you'd like to make it a part of your life.

Use this list to create goals for your plan. Do this exercise at least once a year to ensure your goals and objectives agree with your definition of living healthfully.

Lana's Story

I had a serious bout of pneumonia eighteen years ago. I was told my chances of living were slim if I got it again. Three years ago, I contracted a similar strain. I made it, but not without damage to my right lung. My doctor gave me one word. He said it slowly and very simply—"Move." At first, I thought he meant to pack up and move. *Wrong.* He meant to move my body.

I decided the best way for me to move was to walk. It had to be outside, and it had to be four seasons worth of time. I committed to walk every day before work, five days a week, from 6:00 to 7:00 A.M. On weekends, I would do longer walks on a beautiful river trail or in a preserve. I tried to find charity walks to connect my own philosophy of volunteerism with my commitment to my lung. I seldom spoke of my walks to anyone. I did not care to make it a committee. I am with people all day, and the solitude was a great breeding ground for reflection and prayer.

Soon, I began to notice my clothes were not fitting as they once did. When the size eighteen slipped to a twelve, I went back to my doctor and weighed fifty pounds less. That was one year ago, and I am still fifty pounds less.

The most important lesson I have learned is that it is truly not about weight—not about inches, pounds, calories, carbs, fat grams, or any of the same. I did not visit a scale, nor did I count anything. Most importantly, I did not think in those terms. I never refused myself food I desired. My portions minimized, but it was a natural process. I ate when I was hungry and moving took care of the stress-buster role food used to assume in my life.

Though some need group processing of such an endeavor, I needed the peace my solo flight offered me. I liked the fact that it was *my thing* and in many ways, my secret. I lead a very active lifestyle. I am a high school teacher as well as principal consultant for a Chicago museum. I serve on many boards and have a rigorous speaking career. I knew if I did not walk in the morning, I would not be at the top of my game the rest of the day.

I will never go on a diet again. I am now used to putting on a pair of Gap jeans and not being shocked that they fit, remembering fully the days I would walk by and knew it was not the store for people my size. My stamina is much greater than it used to be and sleep is much more rested. Losing weight on no diet was, is, and will always be a great trail to blaze.

You Can Make a Difference

Think about all you have achieved. Your health, self-esteem, and confidence are now resources you can use to help others meet their health goals. Your capacity to contribute to others' lives has expanded. Take what you learned on your journey to health and help others on their journeys. If you haven't started that support group yet, why not start it now? Find whatever way you can to inspire health and fitness in others.

> *The more you give, the more you will receive. If you want [inspiration], [inspire] others.*
> —Deepak Chopra

It's All About Choices

Every moment of every day, you have the opportunity to choose your response to any situation. Your life is, and will continue to be, the result of your choices. You can make decisions that allow you to grow and move forward, stay where you are, or move backward. You will have great days and not-so-great days ahead. The key is making decisions based upon what you consider most important in your life. When you do that, regardless of what others or your environment dictate, you have made the decision that is right for you.

Books

Body Image

The Body Image Workbook: An 8-Step Program for Learning to Like Your Looks by Thomas F. Cash. Fine Communication: 1998. This book is great for those struggling with their body image. The workbook shows you how to evaluate your body image and how to create a better relationship with your body.

Food and Nutrition

Conscious Cuisine: A New Style of Cooking from the Kitchens of Chef Cary Neff by Cary Neff. Sourcebooks Trade: 2002. This book is perfect for those who already enjoy cooking. Chef Neff makes gourmet meals healthy.

Eat, Drink, and Be Healthy: The Harvard Medical School Guide to Healthy Eating by Walter C. Willett, et al. Free Press: 2002. This is the best book I have read about the connection between what you eat and your health.

Eating Well for Optimum Health: The Essential Guide to Bringing Health and Pleasure Back to Eating by Andrew Weil. Quill: 2001. Dr. Weil clears up the conflicting and confusing information we hear about food and nutrition. His critique of several popular diets, including Atkins, is fantastic.

Food Fight: The Inside Story of the Food Industry, America's Obesity Crisis, and What We Can Do About It by Kelly D. Brownell and Katherine Battle Horgen. McGraw Hill/Contemporary Books: 2003. The authors ask industry, media, and the government to take responsibility for the toxic environment they helped create, while providing useful steps for communities to take action against obesity.

Food Politics: How the Food Industry Influences Nutrition and Health by Marion Nestle. University of California Press: 2003. This book provides a thorough review of the food industry's manipulation of our eating habits and food choices.

Getting Thin and Loving Food: 200 Easy Recipes to Take You Where You Want to Be by Kathleen Daelmans. Houghton Mifflin Co.: 2004. This book combines great, easy recipes with healthful tips and motivational stories.

Taste Pure and Simple: Irresistible Recipes for Good Food and Good Health by Michel Nischan, et al. Chronicle Books: 2003. Delicious recipes from a French chef who changed his cooking after his son was diagnosed with type I diabetes.

General Health

Ageless Body, Timeless Mind by Deepak Chopra. Harmony Books: 1993. Dr. Chopra discusses how important the mind-body connection is in living your best life possible.

Strength Training

Weight Training for Dummies by Liz Neporent and Suzanne Schlosberg. For Dummies: 2000. A great weight-training book for beginners. It includes exercises for each muscle group, descriptions and pictures of proper form, and common mistakes to avoid.

Websites

Athletic Wear

www.athleta.com
www.title9sports.com

Education

www.4woman.gov
The National Women's Health Information Center website provides free, reliable health information for women.

www.healthfinder.gov
This site discusses such topics as prevention of disease, wellness, and alternative medicine.

www.fitness.gov
The President's Council on Physical Fitness.

www.shapeup.org
Learn about portion control, calories, and the latest health research from this site.

www.obesity.org
The American Obesity Organization aims to change public policy and perceptions about obesity. Their site covers such topics as education, research, prevention, treatment, and discrimination of the obese.

www.americanrunning.org
For those interested in running, this is a great site to read up on injury prevention, nutrition, and integration of running into your life.

www.ftc.gov/bcp/conline/edcams/redflag/index.html
A website sponsored by the Federal Trade Commission designed to educate the media and consumers about false claims in advertising diet products. This site provides examples of

the most common false claims used by advertisers, information on how to spot false claims, and a Red Flag Brochure with specific products to avoid.

Events

www.active.com
Search for hundreds of fitness events across the United States.

www.danskin.com/triathlon
This is the site for the Danskin Women's Triathlon, held across the United States every year.

www.ryka.com/events.asp
Go here for more information on Ryka-sponsored women-only events.

www.avonwalk.org
The Avon Walk for Breast Cancer is a great way to get fit while helping fund breast cancer research.

www.komen.org
The Race for the Cure is another way to fund breast cancer research.

www.ava.org
For walkers, the American Volkssport Association provides a list of walking events and clubs in every state.

Exercise

www.jazzercise.com
Yes, Jazzercise still exists. If you're interested in group aerobics classes without having to join a gym, check out this site.

www.videofitness.com
If you're considering using exercise videos, this site gives the advantages and disadvantages of using videos, provides con-

sumer reviews of tapes/DVDs, helps you choose the videos that match your goals, and provides online support.

Food and Nutrition

www.hsph.harvard.edu/nutritionsource
This site, maintained by the Department of Nutrition at the Harvard School of Public Health, covers such topics as food pyramids, fats and cholesterol, exercise, alcohol, fiber, carbohydrates, protein, vitamins, and fruits and vegetables.

www.foodfit.com
This site provides the latest news on healthy eating, cooking, and fitness. If you're looking for healthy recipes, sign up for the free newsletters, "Simply Foodfit" and "Weekend Supper."

Motivation

www.presidentschallenge.org
A physical activity and fitness award program sponsored by the President's Council on Physical Fitness. Register online and track your progress.

www.americaonthemove.org
Challenges you to walk an extra 2,000 steps and eat 100 fewer calories each day. Register and track your progress online.

www.nwcr.ws
The site of the National Weight Control Registry provides the largest collection of weight-loss success stories in the world. The site includes research findings on the eating and exercise habits of successful weight losers. Once you've lost at least thirty pounds and kept it off for a year, you may be eligible to join the registry.

INDEX

I Want to Hear
What You Have to Say

Any and all feedback requested. Please share:
- What you liked about the book
- Any suggestions for improvement
- What you'd like more information about
- Your successes
- Your challenges
- Your story
- Your needs and wants
- *Anything* you want to share

I wrote this book for you. If you have suggestions, *I want to hear them.* Please visit www.trustyourselftotransform.com to provide feedback.

Give the Gift of
Trust Yourself to Transform Your Body
to Your Friends, Family, and Colleagues

ORDER ONLINE AT
www.trustyourselftotransform.com
OR ORDER HERE

❑ **YES**, I want _____ copies of *Trust Yourself to Transform Your Body* at $16.95 each, plus $4.00 shipping for the first book and $2.00 for each additional book (IL residents please add $1.32 sales tax per book). Canadian orders must be accompanied by a postal money order in U.S. funds. Allow 15 days for delivery.

❑ **YES**, I would like *free* information on seminars/workshops.

My check or money order for $_____ is enclosed.

Please charge my: ❑ Visa   ❑ MasterCard
                   ❑ Discover   ❑ American Express

Name _____

Organization _____

Address _____

City/State/Zip _____

Phone_____ E-mail _____

Card # _____

Exp. Date_____ Signature _____

Please make your check payable and return to:
Crimson Leaf Publishing
P.O. Box 7836 • Gurnee, IL 60031

Quantity discounts are available on bulk purchases of this book.